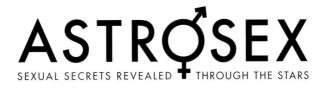

ASTROSEX

SEXUAL SECRETS REVEALED THROUGH THE STARS

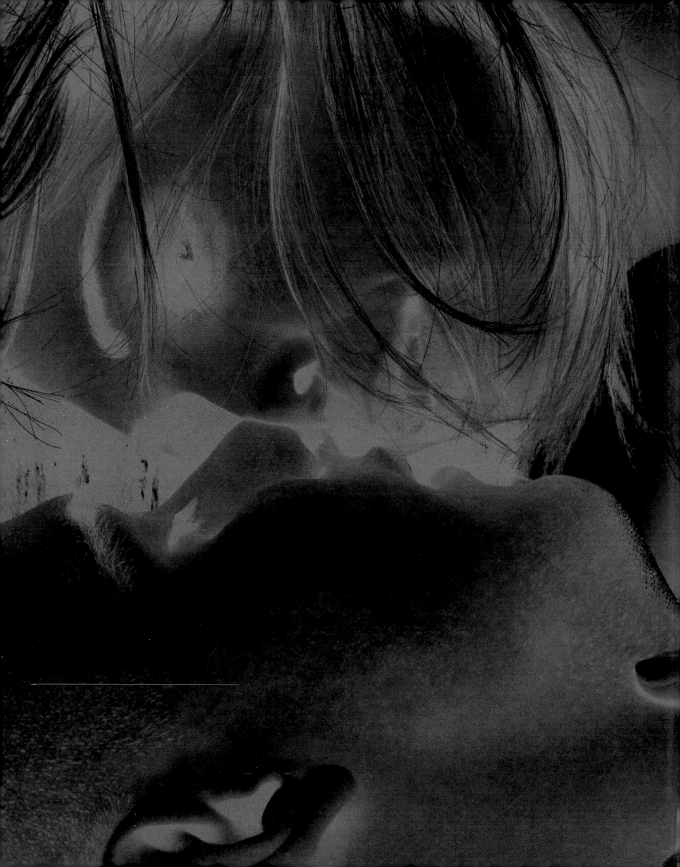

ASTROSEX

SEXUAL SECRETS REVEALED ✛ THROUGH THE STARS

SARAH BARTLETT

SKYHORSE PUBLISHING

Skyhorse Publishing books may be purchased in bulk at
special discounts for sales promotion, corporate gifts,
fund-raising, or educational purposes. Special editions
can also be created to specifications. For details,
contact the Special Sales Department, Skyhorse
Publishing, 307 West 36th Street, 11th Floor, New York,
NY 10018 or info@skyhorsepublishing.com.

Skyhorse® and Skyhorse Publishing® are registered
trademarks of Skyhorse Publishing, Inc.®, a Delaware
corporation.

Visit our website at
www.skyhorsepublishing.com.

10 9 8 7 6 5 4 3 2 1

Library of Congress Cataloging-in-Publication Data is
available on file.

Cover design by Victoria Bellavia

ISBN: 978-1-62914-164-0
E-book ISBN: 978-1-62914-275-3

Printed in Hong Kong

CONTENTS

INTRODUCTION 6

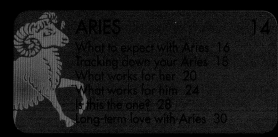

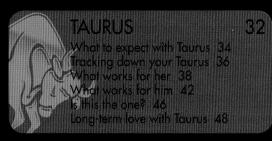

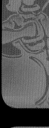
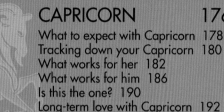
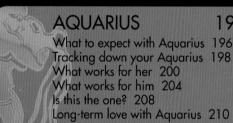
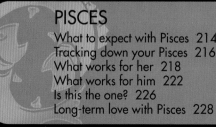

INTRODUCTION

SEXUAL SECRETS

As we are all getting comfortable with the idea that "men are from Mars and women are from Venus," it is worth reminding ourselves that for thousands of years astrologers have been telling us that we are all affected by all of the planets all of the time.

DIFFERENT PATHS

As John Gray's timely treatise *Men Are from Mars, Women Are from Venus* reminds us, our gender has a major influence on our behavior: "Not only do men and women communicate differently but they think, feel, perceive, react, respond, love, need, and appreciate differently." And it's not only our gender that influences our personalities and behavior. Our nationality, culture, upbringing, and social status all have a bearing on the way we feel about ourselves and the way we respond to other people. Even our position within the family unit has an important effect on our relationships (for example, the firstborn of a family of five is usually

responsible and driven while the youngest will be relatively wild and willful). These different factors all serve to modify our behavior and make us unique individuals. Or do they?

THE SAME SIGN

Astrologers believe that regardless of any and all of the factors above, people who are born under any given sign of the zodiac share essentially similar character traits, beliefs, and desires. In essence, they are the same. Detractors (most frequently down-to-earth Capricorns or skeptical Aquarians) are quick to reject astrology on the basis that "no way are one in every twelve of the

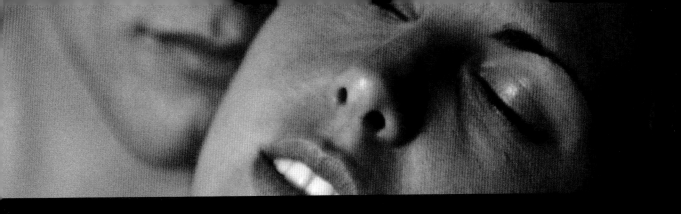

six-and-a-half billion people on Earth the same!"
Again, to a significant extent, yes they are! And is
that really so strange? Modern scientific analysis,
which by definition aims to discredit all things
magical and mystical, has strangely enough led to
a similar conclusion down its own empirical path.
The famous Myers-Briggs psychological profiling
techniques, developed over years of study by
Katharine Cook Briggs and her daughter Isabel
Briggs Myers, drawing on the groundbreaking
work of Dr. Carl Jung, divides us into sixteen
different "types"—that's hardheaded science
stating that one in sixteen of us respond to
circumstances in remarkably similar ways.

A PRACTICAL ART

Those of us who get hooked on astrology begin by
being awed by these similarities and recognizing,
again and again, the influence of the stars on the
lives of those around us, especially in our close
relationships. And, by the way, if a down-to-earth
Capricorn becomes convinced of the practical
use of astrology, there can be no more fervent

advocate of the art. Once hooked, astrology
becomes a way of life and can help us to take
responsibilty for our choices in love and out
of it. It provides a consistent framework for
understanding oneself and others, and is an
endless source of fascination.

Astrology is about bringing out your full potential in life

For most people, sadly, their astrological
adventure begins and ends when they read
their horoscope for the day in their favorite
newspaper, magazine, or website. This is a shame,
because astrology can be so much more than
that. I don't mean that we all have to learn how
to cast a horoscope and interpret birth charts. But
armed with the basics of astrology, every aspect

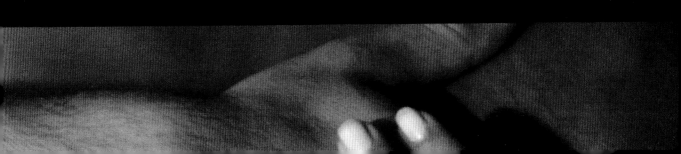

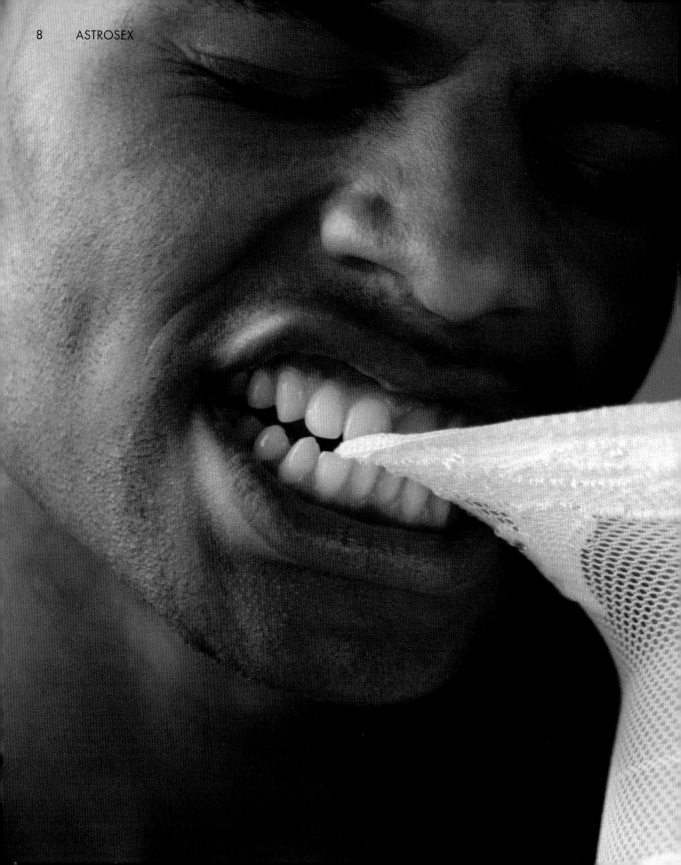

of life can be viewed from a more objective perspective. Understanding the secrets of your sun-sign's qualities (and that of your partner) is a major asset in your love life. When you think about it, our intimate relationships are far and away the most important thing for us all.

NAVIGATE YOUR SEX LIFE VIA THE STARS

Of course, every individual is unique, but we all share many similar qualities and emotions, such as desire, love, hate, anger, and fear. It is how as individuals we express or repress them, or try to compensate for them, that astrology can reveal with such clarity. We all have Venus, Mars, and the rest of the planets in our birth chart exerting their influence to a greater or lesser degree, but in the end it is our sun-sign (also known as our star-sign) that gives the most comprehensive guidance about our sexual preferences, needs, and desires.

Your individual horoscope is a blueprint or map of your psychological makeup. Your sun-sign (the one planetary placement everyone knows) is only one part of your birth chart, but it is the essence of

you. The Sun is the center of our solar system and also at the heart of the astrological chart. In matters of love and sex, your sun-sign (and to a lesser extent the Moon, see pages 236–37) is the all-important signifier. The placement of the Sun at the moment of birth is the key to unlocking the sexual secrets of yourself and others, and represents the core motivation and potential within each of us. By reading this book you can share those secrets. You'll learn what to expect from your partner, what really turns them on, and how to survive long-term love. It also tells you who is compatible with you, and who may pose problems, in bed and out of it.

Perhaps most importantly, your sun-sign also gives you an overview of your own destiny in love, sex, and relationships. Through becoming more aware of who you are, and knowing what works for you and why, you can discover how to deal with your feelings, libido, and sexual needs. Astrology can guide you to understand your own sexual chemistry and to liberate those hidden sexual potentials locked inside you, and with self-awareness you can learn to love more honestly.

ANOTHER PARTNER, ANOTHER PLANET

Why is it that two people can have instant "chemistry," while another two people get together and just seem like a couple of wet blankets? Each zodiac sun-sign lives in a world of its own, and each "thinks, feels, perceives, reacts, responds, loves, needs, and appreciate" in a way that is unique to **that sign.**

ON THE CUSP

The Sun appears to move through each sign of the zodiac throughout the year, spending roughly a month in each sign. Being born on "the cusp" means being born on the day that the sign moves from one zodiac sign to another. There is a common misconception that if you are born on the cusp, or even within a few days on either side of that date, then you may have character traits associated with the "neighboring" sign, as if the journey from Aries Street to Taurus Avenue was a simple matter of stepping across the road. But this is absolutely not the case. You would need a rocket to get from Aries and Taurus—the two signs are worlds apart.

If you were born on the cusp, then remember that you're either one sign or the other; you can't be both. To complicate matters, the Sun changes signs at different time of day depending on the year, and sometimes the day itself changes too. So, if you think you were born on the cusp, you really need to check which sun-sign you are.

PAIRING UP

In relationships we're all searching for something. Some of us dream of merging into a blissful union with our perfect partner, or "soul mate" (no one more than a Pisces), while others just want to merge with as many people as possible in the

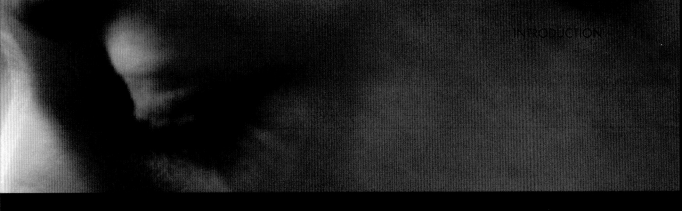

shortest possible time (typical of Sagittarius). Most of us, however, are somewhere in between these two extremes. We want to find Mr. or Miss Right eventually, but we are happy to have a few less-than-perfect partners along the way—especially if the sex is sensational.

But precisely what constitutes "sensational" sex can be drastically different from one sign to another. Each sun-sign's character derives from its ruler. These rulers are the ten planets in the astrological birth chart: Mercury, Venus, Mars, Jupiter, Saturn, Uranus, Neptune, Pluto, and the two luminaries, the Sun and the Moon. Taurus, which is ruled by Venus, the goddess of love, is a true sensualist, wanting classy but steamy arousal and a close, emotional rapport. Taurean bulls know exactly how to turn their partners on, and believe that lovemaking is a work of art. Aries, ruled by Mars, the god of war, is a very different creature: the

ram wants action, challenging fights, and fast and furious sex in adventurous places. Whereas bulls will take time to find out what turns their partners on, rams are impatient, willful, and play games of sexual one-upmanship. And while the indulgent bull prefers the privacy and comfort of his or her own bed, the fiery ram is exciting, dynamic, and adores spontaneous sex in public locations.

So whatever sun-sign you are, the planet that rules that sign is really where you're coming from! In astrological terms, you're only from Mars if you are Aries (whether male or female) and you're only from Venus if you are Taurus or Libra (male or female). If you're Virgo, you're from Mercury; Pisces, you're from Neptune; and so on (see box). These planetary archetypes are at the root of your own sun-sign's expression. Now that you know which planet you're really from, get working on your own personal planet of love and lust as expressed through your personal sun-sign guide. Whether expressing your favorite fantasy or turning your lover on, navigate your love life using all of the planets in the astrological zodiac.

YOUR RULING PLANET

Aries—fiery Mars	Libra—sensual Venus
Taurus—sensual Venus	Scorpio—torrid Pluto
Gemini—suave Mercury	Sagittarius—potent Jupiter
Cancer—subtle Moon	Capricorn—sultry Saturn
Leo—flamboyant Sun	Aquarius—flighty Uranus
Virgo—suave Mercury	Pisces—romantic Neptune

HOW TO USE THIS BOOK

First of all, read the chapter about yourself. No doubt you'll probably see some descriptions and qualities that seem to be spot on, and others that make you raise your hands in horror and think "no, that's not me, how could I be like that?!" But the latter response is very revealing.

We all have a rather biased view of ourselves. There are bits that we like, and bits that we don't like. What usually happens is that we squish, repress, or deny the bits we don't like, or project them onto our lovers. That's when it gets messy. But if you can accept that the shadowy or uncomfortable side of yourself is lurking within, and learn to express it both sexually and emotionally, then you can start to enjoy a much more honest you as well as a more open and honest sexual relationship.

WHERE TO LOOK

If you're single or looking for a new partner, a quick browse through the basic "Star stats" and "What to expect" spreads for the different signs will let you see whether you like the sound of these characters. Alternatively, check the sex grid at the back of the book (pages 230–31) to get a snap evaluation of each combination's relationship potential. Are you turned on by the idea of a fiery, flamboyant Leo, or a stylish but cool Virgo? Which sign do you think would gel with your sexual needs? Perhaps you've already been in a relationship with one or more of these signs, so check out whether they lived up to their reputations, or if they were denying or repressing some of those better qualities.

If attached, you can read the book with your partner. The "What works for her/him" spreads explain how your lover's sun-sign manifests itself in her or his relationship behavior, as well as giving you sex tips and positions that are guaranteed to push all the right astrological buttons. You can dive straight into any of the spreads for sexual guidance, and then check out the "Is this the one?" and "Long-term love" sections to find out just what sort of sexual rapport and relationship you can expect with each sign. Check out both your signs to get to know each other and yourselves a little better, and then enjoy trying out some of the ideas for foreplay, oral sex, turning each other on, and sex-position techniques.

Of course, if you've gotten to the end of a section and decided that your double-the-fun Gemini is too much of a handful or your clingy Cancer crab is becoming a drag, the last page also points you to the easy way out of the relationship with the lowdown on exactly what moves to make to get yourself shown the exit in short order.

This book is a sexual indulgence, and, of course, you can always read it alone and enjoy it for its erotic, raunchy content. But whether sexually a twosome or alone and loving it, this book will reveal more about you and your partner than you could ever possibly imagine. Enjoy.

sexual preferences by reading the sex-position boxes and "How to make her/him horny" sections for the other signs in the same element as yours or your partner's.

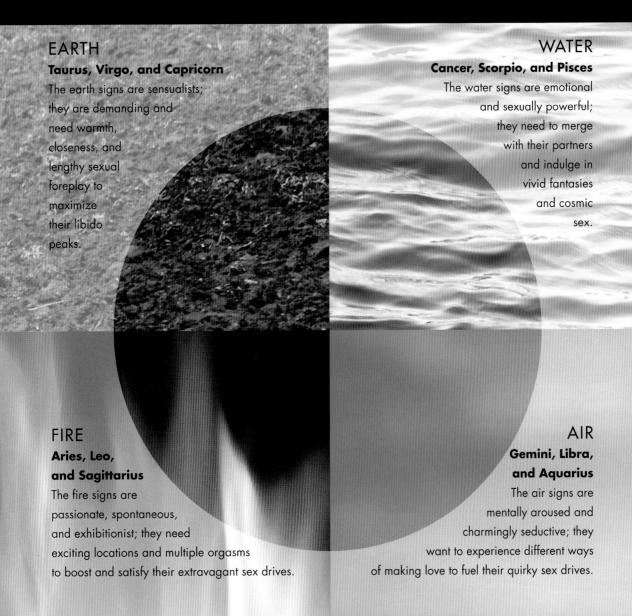

EARTH
Taurus, Virgo, and Capricorn
The earth signs are sensualists; they are demanding and need warmth, closeness, and lengthy sexual foreplay to maximize their libido peaks.

WATER
Cancer, Scorpio, and Pisces
The water signs are emotional and sexually powerful; they need to merge with their partners and indulge in vivid fantasies and cosmic sex.

FIRE
Aries, Leo, and Sagittarius
The fire signs are passionate, spontaneous, and exhibitionist; they need exciting locations and multiple orgasms to boost and satisfy their extravagant sex drives.

AIR
Gemini, Libra, and Aquarius
The air signs are mentally aroused and charmingly seductive; they want to experience different ways of making love to fuel their quirky sex drives.

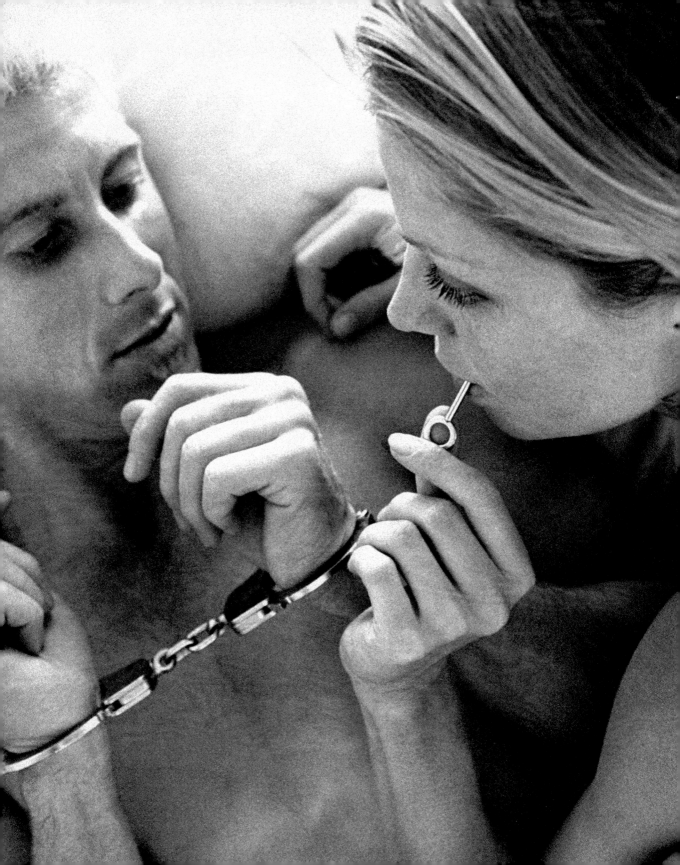

ARIES
MARCH 21 — APRIL 20

STAR STATS

Ruling planet MARS
Signature symbol THE RAM
Metal IRON
Stone RUBY
Color SCARLET

Where to find Aries At any sport's venue, cruising the casino, or working out at the gym.

Hot date Aries adore action. Go to a cross-country rally, the nearest roller coaster ride, or adventure park. Or invite Aries to try a bungee jump!

Needs and desires Competitive, feisty, and impulsive, Aries needs to be the center of adoring attention. But a provocative lover is also a must.

Top turn-on Erotic fiction, oral sex in the car, and spontaneous sex outdoors.

Sex positions The Eagle
 Potent Penetration

Sex toy Peaches, grapes, lickable juicy fruit.

Sex statistic 89 percent of Arians are competitive about their sexual performance.

WHAT TO EXPECT WITH ARIES

Feisty Aries is goal oriented and aggressive. Impulsive at worst and daredevil at best, this is one outgoing, impatient sign. Rams have to be first in everything. First to arrive on the date and first to orgasm. Arians want it all, now. Volatile and daring, their libidos are set to red alert and they love a sexual challenge.

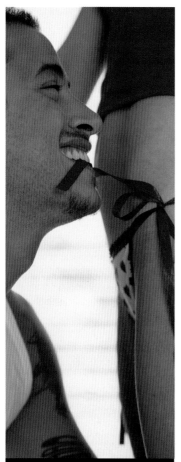

PULLING THE STRINGS
Assertive and strong-willed, Aries likes to take the lead in the bedroom, whether by direct action or by giving the orders.

Action-packed Arians are ruled by Mars, the god of war. And it's not surprising that they are renowned for being pushy, feisty, and overconfident. This rubs off on their relationships, of course. If you can keep up with them—or at least keep them chasing after you—then they might find time to stop and get to know you better. The main problem is that they are so interested in themselves, what they are going to do tomorrow and how they are going to right all the wrongs in the world, that you have to accept you're going to play second fiddle to this first violin.

SEX BOMBS

Rams pride themselves on being walking sex bombs. And they do make formidable lovers. Provocative and fiery in bed, they're impulsive, charismatic romantics who want action and drama in all aspects of their life. Although they love to show off their sexual know-how, they won't be particularly interested in whether they're making the earth move for you too. However, if you're assertive about your own sexual turn-ons, then they'll rise to the occasion in true crusading style.

CHILD'S PLAY

For all their dramatic self-will, the ram is a child at heart. They need adventure, the space to express their temper, and a partner who is as independent and spirited as they are. If you're an easy catch, they probably won't even bother, and if you don't enthuse about their latest crusade or the Harley Davidson bike parked up the road, they'll be off in search of an equal. But if you can match up to them for courage, challenge, and personal freedom, they might just hang around with you rather than hang glide off into the sunset.

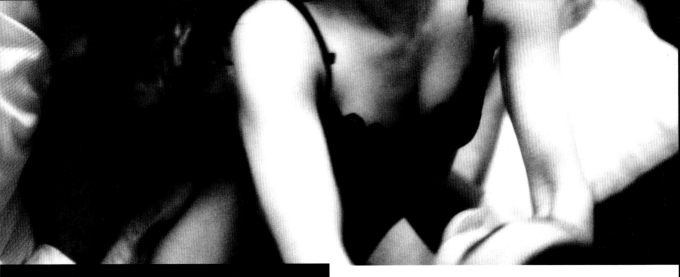

THE ARIES MAN

Aries is the first masculine sign of the zodiac, self-willed and warrior-like. He adores chasing, hunting, and being challenged. And if you let him get too close to you too soon, the chances are he'll feel it's all too easy, so why bother? The ram is motivated by desire. He lives and breathes it, rarely letting anything get in the way of his single-minded vision. And because he must be always on a quest, you'll have to either be tantalizingly unavailable or give him a marathon-like run for his money. This macho, self-made man is often accused of egotism. He knows that his purpose in life is to prove to the world and to himself that he's a hero and a sex god. He's looking for an extraordinary woman who can be as independent and adoring as he is, who can keep up with all his appetites, and who will join in all those physical sports—like sex!

THE ARIES WOMAN

Miss Aries is one determined heroine. This hot-headed, independent lady needs challenge and romance 24/7. When you do get hunted down by her, you'll quickly realize that you're in competition

> In the **battle of the sexes** she aims to be **one-up** on her man.

with her, both intellectually and in bed. But her greatest qualities shine through if you treat her as an equal. She's sexy, romantic, self-willed, and vain. Give her bags of space, be as adventurous as she is, and you'll have the opportunity to be with one very special and exciting woman.

ARIES IN A NUTSHELL

KEYWORDS Irrepressible; impatient; fiery; driven; courageous; challenging; lusty; idealistic; insensitive

LIKES Freedom; competition; being in love; showing off; one-upmanship

DISLIKES Routine sex; not getting his or her way; wimps; being told to wait (for anything!)

TRACKING DOWN YOUR ARIES

Fast-paced Arians aren't the easiest of zodiac signs to track down. Their love of thrills and spills, adventure and action, means they won't hang around in one place for long. But if you're up for competition, sport, and risks, you might be lucky enough to get hunted out yourself.

Arians are always just in one big hurry everywhere they go. In fact, if they're not racing fast cars or grabbing a coffee on the run, then they'll be the ones elbowing their way to the head of a line, just to prove that they're leader of the pack. Hard-working and energetic, they're willing to take risks most people wouldn't dream of, and are brilliant at inventing new ways of doing traditional things, whether in politics or business.

EXTREME SPORTS
The thing about Arians is that they prefer tracking you down.

Although this is a highly sexed sign, Aries prefers to be chaste rather than chased. So it simply pays to be in the right environment, and with luck, you'll have to make a run for it and let them hunt you out. Their innate love of action and adventure means they take to extreme sports like fish to water. If you're prepared to be a daredevil bungee jumper, surfer, skydiver, or rock climber, then the chances are you'll be desirable. You're far more likely to find Aries hanging out in a fast-food diner than a six-course gourmet restaurant. They just don't have the patience.

> Arians live life in the fast lane, so you'll have to be quick off the mark if you want to attract their attention

Check out sports shops too. They love trying out all that sporty stuff.

MENTAL CHALLENGE

Not all Arians are up for physical competitiveness. There are many who adore intellectual challenges instead. They make great artists, philosophers, visionaries, and gurus. With their love of fighting on behalf of the underdog, you'll also find them in top positions in the legal profession. In fact, they adore all the theater of the courtroom and will rise dynamically to the challenge of winning a legal case.

Outdoor-loving, active Arians are very rarely at home for long: they'd rather be jogging around the park, jumping on a bike, or tearing around town painting it red—Anything that satisfies their need for action, thrills, and fast-paced competition. Be one step ahead and the ram will be ready for a new challenge: you.

PLACES TO LOOK

THE DANCE FLOOR

Fiery Aries can't resist throwing themselves about in a nightclub. As long as they can lead the dance, you might find they lead you on to sexier things too.

SPORTY VENUES

Whether it's a grand-prix race or a surfers' beach, the ram loves action sports. Cheer at the checkered flag or ride the waves, and you might just get spotted.

POLITICAL DEBATES

Get down to your local public meetings and watch flamboyant Aries stirred into saving the town from oppressors and bureaucrats.

SANDWICH BARS

Watch for the ones who dive in and out quickly. Bump into them as if by chance, flash a sexy smile, and wait to be pursued.

ARIES TOP TEN CAREERS

1 Headhunter
2 Company director
3 Barrister
4 Solicitor
5 Financial advisor
6 Sports teacher
7 Politician
8 Art director
9 Firefighter
10 Ambulance driver

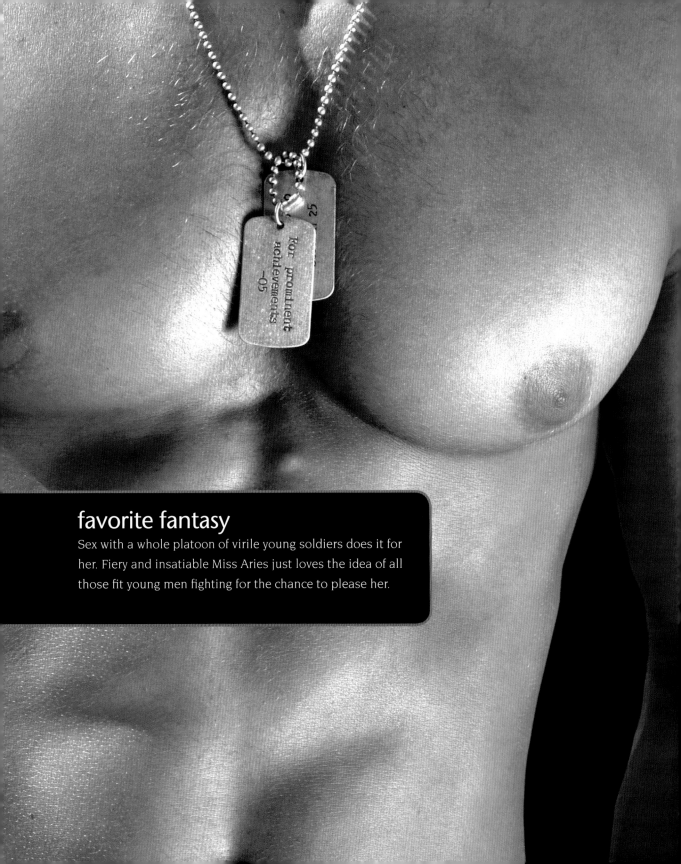

favorite fantasy

Sex with a whole platoon of virile young soldiers does it for
her. Fiery and insatiable Miss Aries just loves the idea of all
those fit young men fighting for the chance to please her.

WHAT WORKS FOR HER

The ultimate huntress, the Aries woman just won't take no for an answer. Romantic and feisty, she's happy to sweep a man off his feet and is challenging and competitive in the bedroom. That's why she's looking for a lover who not only can match her for spirit but also respects her need for independence.

It's the hunt and sexual conquest that turns the Aries woman on, just as much as all the steamy action. In fact, if she's ignored or rejected, the ram is even more determined to have you. And she will. Fiery Aries thrives on challenging, adrenaline-racing relationships, with men who are equally hot-headed, impulsive, and potent. She's looking for someone who accepts her need to be first in everything, whether it is first in the shower or the first to win a game of strip poker. When she says she wants sex now, she means now, not

> You must be able to **match** her fire and drive **between the sheets** and be ready for **sexy antics** at a moment's notice

later. At parties she's one of the biggest flirts around, and she'll make the decision about which lucky contender is going to be blessed with her sexy company.

EXCITING

There are times when Aries can be a tad reckless, leaping into someone's bed without caring if he's already dating or attached. Ruled by impatient Mars, she needs her independence and also a man who's a bit of a local hero and can make her sex life glamorous and stimulating. She needs the buzz of change and excitement, not routine.

HOW TO MAKE HER HORNY

The Aries woman's prime astro-erogenous zone begins at the tip of her earlobes, extending all around her face, toward her eyes, and then up across her forehead. Traditionally, Aries rules the head, so start off by nibbling or gently biting her earlobes. Next tongue and caress her earlobes,

push your tongue a little into her ear and then whisper your favorite erotic fantasy. Next trace your fingers across her face, along the lines of her cheeks and down her nose. Now you've got to speed things up a little, or she'll get bored, so kneel or stand above her and rub your penis across her temples to give her a real adrenaline surge, and let the battle commence.

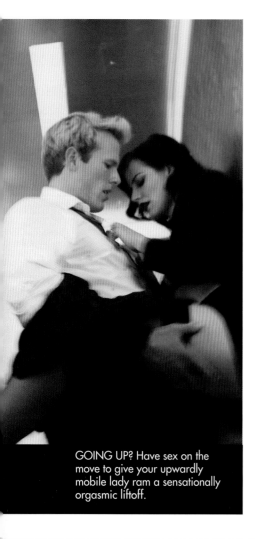

GOING UP? Have sex on the move to give your upwardly mobile lady ram a sensationally orgasmic liftoff.

COMPETITIVE URGE

Aries really thrives with a partner who'll compete with her for who's going to be on top in bed, or who just adores having pillowfights. Danger and excitement also contribute to her adrenaline surges. She's likely to ask for sex at any moment of the day when the feeling comes over her. Slow, sensual foreplay isn't for Aries. She just wants to get on with it and climax over and over again. It's fast and feisty penetration that electrifies her the most. The more imaginative and challenging you are, the more aroused she'll get.

OUT AND ABOUT

Sex in daylight is a real turn-on, especially if she pretends you're a stranger she's just met. Try public locations: on the airplane, in the shopping mall, anywhere that you can "nearly" make an exhibition of yourselves. The more likely you are to be caught, the better her orgasm. Aries is one of the connoisseurs of sex on the move. She'll adore fondling your penis in the car when the traffic lights are red. Mirrors, saucy videos, and erotic movies are among her greatest turn-ons, and your ram will be in sexual nirvana watching herself having sex in front of a mirror, or sharing mutual masturbation while watching a porn movie.

FAST AND FABULOUS

Electrifying, demanding, and provocative, Aries loves to set the pace, to dominate, and to challenge. She prefers fast, hard stimulation to slow, sensual indulgence. And when she really gives her all, she turns into a real tigress. Talk dirty in her ear, your tongue licking her hard

THE EAGLE

Passionate about potent and powerful penetration, the Eagle position is perfect for the Aries woman. She loves to take the sexual initiative and the Eagle enables her to control the pace and be on top. You lie on the floor or bed and ask her to stand above and astride you. This initial visual stimulation will give you both a powerful adrenaline rush, setting the mood for the ram to dominate.

LET ARIES KNEEL ASTRIDE YOU, guiding you powerfully into her vagina. This means she can control the force and thrust of deep penetration and still feel in command.

HER TOP TURNOFFS

PREDATORS
She needs to act out the part of a huntress, not someone else's prey.

GAMES
If you're out to catch yourself a ram, don't be sheepish! If you aren't direct and honest, or don't know how to ask for sex directly, then get out quick.

ORDINARY LIFESTYLE
If you've got one, don't reveal it. Pretend to be a racing driver, but never say you're an accountant. She needs to live on the wild side.

WIMPS
Weak willed or lazy? Forget it. And who needs a mother figure when you could have a warrior queen?

ROUTINE SEX
What more can I say?

against her neck for instant arousal. Her quick responses and multiple orgasms mean she often won't wait for you to come. And she won't be slowed down by anybody.

Aries is secretly in need of sexual freedom, so she can resort to having sex for the sake of sex, and often sleeps around. Her biggest challenge is learning to accept that her man isn't just a rival to be beaten on an intimate basis. She needs to learn to let go and at times let you take control so that she can liberate her vulnerable feminine soul, rather than merely act out the dominatrix. Don't forget that Aries is passionate, erotic, and a secret romantic. An attention seeker, if she feels insecure she can get jealous. Most of all, love her for the moment. Don't ask about commitment, and make sure you stay independent and

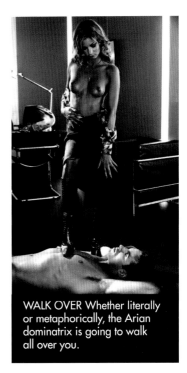

WALK OVER Whether literally or metaphorically, the Arian dominatrix is going to walk all over you.

very hard to catch. Sexual exclusivity is not in the Aries vocabulary, so don't expect too much too soon. But match her for sexual potency, and she might just stick around for longer than she intended.

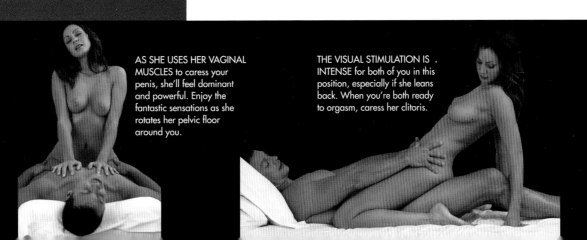

AS SHE USES HER VAGINAL MUSCLES to caress your penis, she'll feel dominant and powerful. Enjoy the fantastic sensations as she rotates her pelvic floor around you.

THE VISUAL STIMULATION IS . INTENSE for both of you in this position, especially if she leans back. When you're both ready to orgasm, caress her clitoris.

WHAT WORKS FOR HIM

This is one ramrod of a sign both physically and mentally. In fact, the Aries man is on a mission: he has a goal, and that's to prove that he's not only a hero, but also God's gift to women. With an extraordinary libido and competitive sex drive, he needs an extraordinary woman to match.

> He loves to **change** romantic **tactics**: be as passionate about the game of **romance** as he is

The Aries man is a bit of a male chauvinist. He's also an idealist when it comes to himself and his perception of women. He's the ultimate masculine hero: lusty and as feisty as the god of war—Mars himself—and that's that. With so much self-interest, he does forget that women have feelings and are not all sex goddesses or princesses in the tower who need rescuing. Aries has trouble "seeing" the woman he's with instead of the ideal of his dreams. Yet this exciting but rather emotionally blinkered rogue is challenging in bed, and most of all passionate about life. If you can match him for sexual stamina, and identify with that fire queen image he has of you, then you'll have a true hero by your side.

WOLF IN RAM'S CLOTHING

One of the ram's best qualities is his incredible desire for change and romance. He's a sexual hunter, but he also likes elusive, uncatchable women. The paradox is, of course, how can you be both? Dress like a vamp, but be totally feminine. Flirt with his friends, but flatter him and boost his ego with the odd sexual innuendo. Most of all, be his equal and have your own life.

HOW TO MAKE HIM HORNY

They say Aries men have erections 70 percent of the time (and that includes when asleep), so it might come as a surprise to you that he's pretty vulnerable in the sexual relationship department. This is because he's not truly in touch with the sensual and emotional side of himself and is more concerned with living up to his macho image than worrying about his partner's sexual needs. However, the ram's astro-erogenous zone is centered around his head and face, and even if he's impatient for penetration, keep him on red alert by tonguing his lips, face, and eyelids. Lick his cheeks, then kiss him deeply, tongue in throat. Whisper erotic fantasies in his ear, and sit astride his torso and push your pelvic floor hard against him, then move up over his face and let him lick your clitoris—he'll be hotter than a fresh baguette!

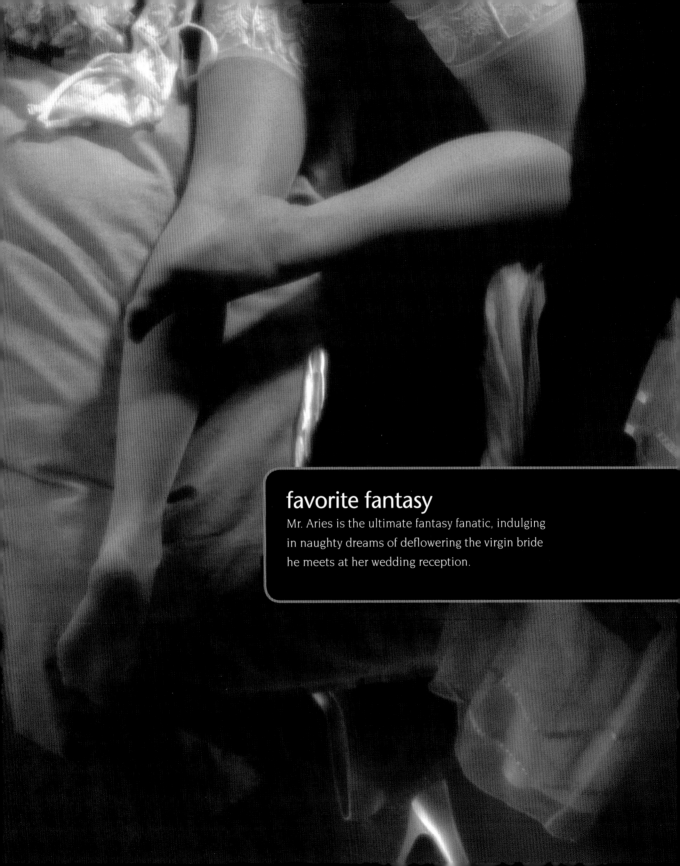

favorite fantasy

Mr. Aries is the ultimate fantasy fanatic, indulging in naughty dreams of deflowering the virgin bride he meets at her wedding reception.

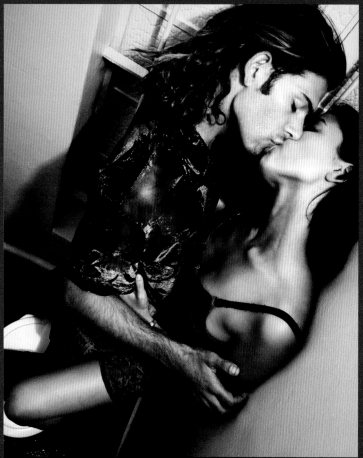

STANDING OVATION The spontaneous and risk-taking ram is always up for quickies in public locations where you might just get caught.

CASANOVA

Aries isn't particularly known for being monogamous when young. He's desperately trying to prove to himself and to everyone around him that he's Mr. Potency. And he's easily led astray by anyone who takes his fancy. In fact, his reputation as a bit of a Casanova ironically stems from his fear of getting too close, because his "ideal woman" hardly ever matches up to the reality, so he's off to make another sexual conquest. In a way, Aries is eternally running away from himself. Emotionally vulnerable, he gets off on spontaneous sex, hard penetration, and quick orgasm because it means he doesn't have to "feel" anything. The ram believes he's the ultimate stud and he'll even play a part in a porno film for the turn-on, just to show off his penis power.

POTENT PENETRATION

He's quickly aroused by taking a dominant position, and his primitive approach to sex is all about action, more action, and few words. Oral sex is a great taster, but it's fast and furious penetration, and lots of it, that gives him the most pleasure. His stamina is incredible, so opt for a position where he has maximum visual stimulation and can literally bang away for hours, changing position to suit you too.

START BY LYING at the edge of a table or bed: he stands or kneels in front of you and you stroke his chest with your feet, or rest them on his shoulders. Let him thrust as deeply as he wants.

TAKING RISKS

Spontaneous seduction gives him instant adrenaline surges. He's aroused by adventure, power, and danger tinged with the unknown. He's turned on by a woman who takes the lead and then submits. So seduce him in a "nearly" public place when he least expects it and then let him take over. His sexual arousal is instant if you act like danger woman, drag him to the party cloakroom or behind the shed and then submit to hard and fast penetration. Suggest having sex in the elevator with him—it's one of his favorite erotic danger haunts—then push up against his buttocks, or naughtily tease his testicles with your fingers when the elevator full of people

EXHIBITIONIST

Quickies and oral sex in public locations give him an instant thrill. Make love standing in front of a mirror or by an open window in daylight, if you dare. He's turned on by exhibitionism try the parking lot or lay-by. The more public and daring, the lengthier his orgasm. Take the initiative and tell him over a romantic dinner that you want sex with him in the bathroom, now!

HONEST INJUN

Aries needs to learn to let his partner make a few of the sex decisions sometimes. But most of all, he needs to acknowledge his own fear of intimacy and his need for constant change. Aries is one of the most testosterone-driven lovers of the zodiac, and his need for quick orgasmic release often means he's ahead of his partner in the arousal stakes. This can create a lack of mutual satisfaction if you aren't assertive about your needs.

HIS TOP TURNOFFS

POSSESSIVENESS

Never assume he's yours for life, or he'll ram you out of his. Keep your independence.

REALITY CHECKS

Tell him that knights in shining armor don't exist and you're in big trouble. Support his romantic dreams.

ROUTINE

Woe betide if you're up for routine sex: Aries prefers improvisation. Make sure you're a sexual pioneer, not a sexual has-been.

BOSSY BOOTS

Don't ever boss him around. Even if he's left his smelly socks on the floor, never tell him to pick them up, or battle will commence.

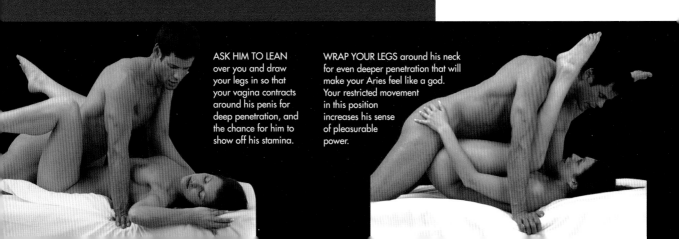

ASK HIM TO LEAN over you and draw your legs in so that your vagina contracts around his penis for deep penetration, and the chance for him to show off his stamina.

WRAP YOUR LEGS around his neck for even deeper penetration that will make your Aries feel like a god. Your restricted movement in this position increases his sense of pleasurable power.

IS THIS THE ONE?

Fiery and energetic, rams are looking for someone who won't tie them down to the boring reality of life. If you can spend every day as if it were a grand-prix race outing, then maybe you'll still be together beyond the checkered flag.

ARIES AND ARIES

Powerful rapport, but who's going to be the boss? You're both vain, impulsive, and argumentative. Could be an exciting sparring match, and neither will feel resentment toward the other if you part. Sexy, but volatile and unstable.

TAURUS AND ARIES

Aries is forever on the go, while Taurus would rather flop around on the sofa, but you are fascinated by your very differences. You'll share anything, but Taurus is likely to fall asleep just when Aries is ready for more.

GEMINI AND ARIES

Fantastic physical bond. Gemini adores the ram's fiery, sexual dynamism, but Aries is self-centered and demanding. Usually passionate, but draining. The twins' desire to outsmart Aries is likely to get them rammed out in the end.

CANCER AND ARIES

Excellent for a short-term affair, but Aries will tire of the crab's roundabout approach to life, when he or she'd rather just get on with it. Words like commitment and security send the ram running, and the crab's clinginess will drive Aries mad.

LEO AND ARIES

Expect to get on like a house on fire. Flames of passion make for a provocative rapport. But proud Leo hates the way Aries flirts in public. Good for a glamorous, sexy partnership, but can burn itself out equally fast.

VIRGO AND ARIES

Very much an attraction of contrasting types, and could be a very steamy romance if Virgo can cope with the ram's extrovert personality. However, can Aries put up with Virgo's need for sex in private?

Natural opposites of the zodiac and, like any polarity, can be a knock-out relationship. Your attraction is immediate and romantic. Aries love to be in charge; Librans love decisions to be made for them. Always fascinating, seldom forgettable.

LIBRA AND ARIES

A very deep and intense sexual relationship, bewitching each other by your very different natures. However, Scorpio is all or nothing, and Aries fights against giving up independence. Be prepared for a long haul of emotional battles.

SCORPIO AND ARIES

Sex is one big adventure for you two. But both of you have a habit of disappearing at a moment's notice. Good for laughs and sexual romps, but be prepared to cross canyons to find each other when you're both off flirting with life.

SAGITTARIUS AND ARIES

A battle of wills, but a physical magnetism. Aries loves taking risks, and initially this will goad the more sexually conventional goat. But Capricorn prefers the kind of risks that lead to business success rather than simply to bed.

CAPRICORN AND ARIES

Both need lots of freedom, but have very different outlooks on love. Aquarius is a thinker, Aries a doer. Sexually, Aries is hot, while Aquarius can seem cool. A great open relationship, but Aquarius could irritate the ram with intellectual superiority.

AQUARIUS AND ARIES

Passionate and audacious, Aries can't resist the fish's romanticism. Pisces easily surrenders to Aries' games and uninhibited sexuality. Difficult when Pisces needs to feel totally part of the ram's life, while Aries wants to be a lone wolf.

PISCES AND ARIES

AND THE WINNER IS...

Aries is not an easy sign for long-term love. But when rams do realize that freedom and commitment are not mutually exclusive, they can find physical and romantic fulfillment with the other fire signs, Leo and Sagittarius. The only sign that can truly give Arians a run for their money, however, is Libra. The ram's need for larger-than-life action is fueled by Libra's own love of personal space. Both idealists, they'll discover sizzling sex and an easy-going, unemotional romantic partnership.

LONG-TERM LOVE WITH ARIES

Arians need lights, camera, action, and drama in their lives. And they do like to be the boss, both around the home and in bed. But if you are truly enthusiastic about everything they do and enjoy the odd healthy expression of anger and love to get out and about, then Aries makes one of the most dynamic and loyal of lovers you can find.

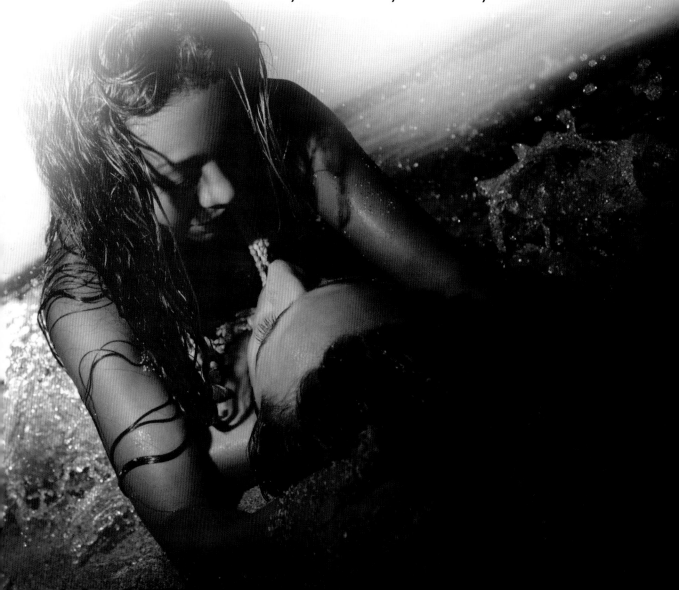

With the ram's love of all things physical, make sure you are prepared for an active lifestyle. If you can't keep up with your partner, at least be there at the finish line cheering him or her on, otherwise your Aries will be off. Be willing to compete with your ram in any mental challenge. But remember that rams don't want an easy pushover; they want to win you over. So accept that you'll eventually have to compromise or give way, even

Aries that he or she is simply the best in everything he or she does. Give unstinting reassurance and support about his or her leadership potential, and he or she'll return the favor tenfold.

RAM BEAU

Rams are essentially children at heart, throwing themselves into missions left, right, and center, burning the candles at both ends and thriving on a

> The **flamboyant** Arian has a **vulnerable** side as well. If you are **supportive**, you'll reap the reward of a very **sexy** partnership.

if you know you were right all along—because, I'm afraid, Aries knows best. Let the ram win, and you'll win that fiery heart too.

FEEL-GOOD FACTOR

Arians need to have constant reassurance that they are the "greatest of them all". This is one very insecure sign at heart, which is why rams compensate by being show-offs, leaders, and fiery protagonists. Tell your

colorful, active, and romantic life. Give them oodles of encouragement, support their dreams and fantasies, however impractical they seem, and they'll reward you by being the most generous, fun-loving, and exciting partners around. And if you understand that underneath that energetic and trail-blazing approach to life lies a very soft heart, then your future together looks red hot and very, very rosy.

LOSING YOUR SHEEP

Rams never think about the practicalities of life—that's someone else's problem—and they certainly can't bear to be ordered around. So the best strategy for getting Arians to dump you is to tell them it's time they did a spot of tidying up. Then leave dirty clothes in heaps on the floor, dirty dishes strewn around the kitchen, and you'll drive Aries right up the wall and right out of your life. These perfectionists can't bear sloppiness, and if you let your standards slide, you can kiss good-bye to your Aries.

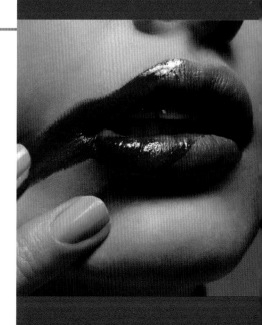

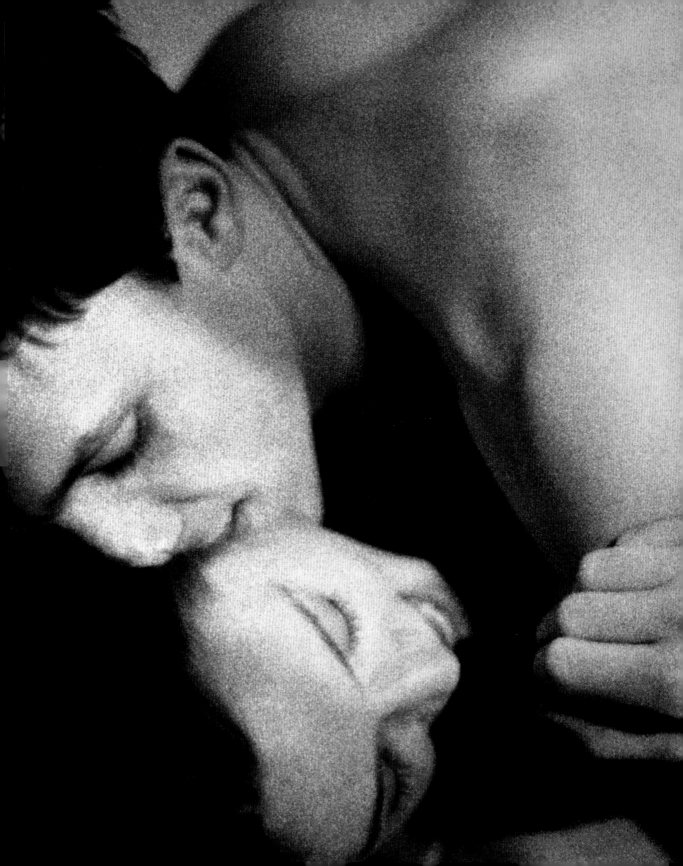

TAURUS

APRIL 21 — MAY 21

STAR STATS

Ruling planet VENUS
Signature symbol THE BULL
Metal COPPER
Stone EMERALD
Color SHOCKING PINK

Where to find Taurus Tracking down the latest designer fashions in the best part of town.

Hot date Take Taurus to the best restaurant in town with the most expensive wine list! Taurus likes to be wined and dined.

Needs and desires Stubborn, sensual, loyal Taurus needs stability, sex—lots of it—and an equally devoted mate.

Top turn-on Silk sheets, silk underwear, and silk pyjamas (preferably on the bedroom floor!).

Sex positions ♀ Mission Accomplished
♂ Man on a Mission

Sex toy An erotic massager.

Sex statistic 79 percent of Taureans own a vibrator—yes, the men too!

WHAT TO EXPECT WITH TAURUS

Sensual Taurus enjoys nothing more than the physical pleasures in life: good food, good wine, good sex. But the bull has a tendency to overindulge, especially when it comes to material possessions. This lover of beauty is, however, one of the most affectionate and reliable signs of the zodiac.

Taurus is ruled by Venus, the goddess of love, beauty, sex, and, don't forget, vanity. The sexiness of Taureans isn't just about what they get up to in bed. It exudes from the way they dress, their body language, and their social interaction. Taureans are pros in the art of passive seduction and are often wicked flirts. But once they fall in love they won't easily fall out. Sexually, be prepared to give your all to a Taurus—a dissatisfied bull has few qualms about looking elsewhere for complete fulfillment.

SLOW AND SENSUAL

Stability and security may be crucial for Taurus in a long-term relationship, but you'll never have a dull or boring sex life. Taureans take a down-to-earth approach to sex and are known for being generous, sensitive, and understanding lovers. They treat making love as a work of art and are never happier than when making their partners happy. Their straightforward nature is a bonus, because they know exactly what they want and they're not afraid to ask for it. Quality sex is what Taureans offer, and they demand it back too.

LOYAL LOVERS

If you want a faithful lover, then seek out a Taurus. But take care not to cross a bull. They will never forgive you, particularly if you cheat on them. But if you are as loyal and true as they are, then they'll always be there for you, both as a friend and lover. Also, watch out for fireworks if you're the argumentative type: bulls have short fuses and will stubbornly believe that they are always right. You'll find they can get fanatical about anything from the spot on your chin to their own sexual prowess.

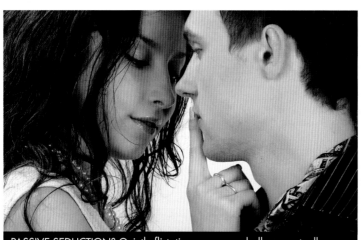

PASSIVE SEDUCTION? Quietly flirtatious, sensuous bulls are actually upfront and wicked about exactly what they want.

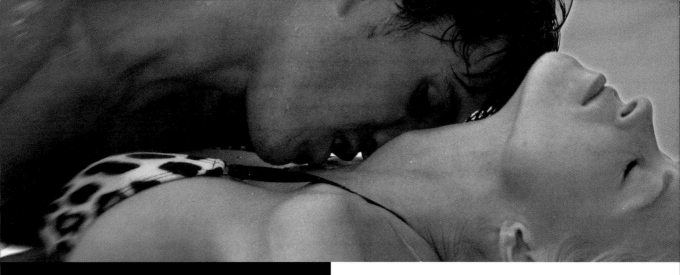

THE TAURUS MAN

The Taurus man can be a sexual conquistador, but he's really searching for a long-lasting, committed love affair. It's in his nature to thoroughly indulge himself in sensual pleasure, but for all his earthy, practical approach to life, he's an utter romantic. Spoil him with gifts, wear beautiful perfume, but remember he has a macho streak, and he will treat *you* like one of his possessions too. He's unlikely to make the first move in the love game, mainly because he wants you to seduce him so he doesn't make a fool of himself (he fears rejection). He'll also want you to take the initiative in bed, except when he's in a monopolizing mood—expect sparks if you're a fiery dominatrix! Taurus is the ultimate strong, silent type, and he'll want to bring you to a climax over and over again. He loves to prove he's the sexiest and most generous of signs.

THE TAURUS WOMAN

This Venus-ruled woman is looking for stability and sexual pleasure. She's sensual, romantic, down-to-earth, and often a little vain. And she's all woman. She's utterly feminine and will give her heart to the

> She might **flirt with your friends**, but it's just a **bit of fun**

one she adores. But she needs a devoted lover to treat her like a lady and seduce her conventionally. Attracted to money, class, beautiful clothes, and men with sexy voices, she's often in demand and hard to catch, but when you do, she'll be there forever.

TAURUS IN A NUTSHELL

KEYWORDS Sensual; loyal; down-to-earth; reliable; vain; affectionate; possessive; jealous; determined; stable; creative

LIKES Feeling secure; being pampered; commitment; beautiful objects and people

DISLIKES Empty promises; being rushed; being told what to do; small portions of food

TRACKING DOWN YOUR TAURUS

Taurus isn't difficult to track down. Bulls won't outrun you like flighty Geminis, or outsmart you like clever Aquarians. They tend to invest a lot of time and energy in their homes and appearances and resent too much change. They love shopping, eating out at the best restaurants, and being at one with nature.

Taurus is a true lover of luxury. And money. Material acquisitions help create a feeling of worth— an outward sign of the bull's achievements. Taureans are either cautious with their cash or extravagant. However, they do believe you have to speculate to accumulate. This abiding interest in money isn't only emotional. Bulls are practical about their finances and suit money-making careers like banking, insurance, and the stock exchange. But take care: Taureans are quite capable of selling out on their own values for something they think is worth more.

A FINE ART

Taureans' appreciation of beauty and their desire to indulge in the finer things of life inevitably lead them to the finest places. You're more likely to find your bull hanging out in swanky designer shops than at the car boot sale. Taurus enjoys beauty in many forms, particularly art and music, and they often have a talent in one or both of these areas. Taurus also rules the throat, and they're blessed with attractive, resonant speaking or singing voices. Bulls are hard workers as well. They have great tenacity, and will stick with

Whether they're in the **town or country**, you'll find **earthy** Taureans in pursuits that **indulge** their **sensuous side**

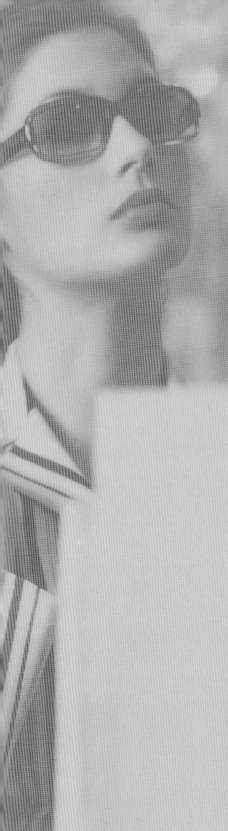

projects with which others have long since lost patience.

AT ONE WITH NATURE

Tickle a bull with a blade of grass and he or she is in heaven. Whether they're watching a sunset or digging their garden, it's communing with nature that makes Taureans feel good to be alive. They are crazy about planting things and watching them grow. Real down-to-earth homemakers, Taureans love to create their very own private Garden of Eden. And as much as they adore their homes, on the weekend you're bound to spot them outdoors hiking across the countryside admiring the landscape, creating spectacular rose gardens in waste ground, or just picnicking in the park. With a deep-seated awareness of the rhythms of nature, no other sign in the zodiac is closer to the earth itself than Taurus.

PLACES TO LOOK

TOP DESIGNER STORES

If the price is high, it must be good. No outrageous fashions, but silk underwear is a must.

PERFUMERY

Sensual Taurus knows the impact of smell. They maximize their allure with seductive, expensive scents.

BEST RESTAURANTS

Fine food and wine satisfy the bull. But they need to watch their tendency to pile on the pounds!

HOME IMPROVEMENT STORES

Taureans love DIY-ing around the home. They have a talent for making their lovenest the most romantic place on earth.

THE KITCHEN

If they're not eating food, then they're cooking it. Taurus often makes a brilliant chef.

TAURUS TOP TEN CAREERS

1 Financial advisor
2 Investment banker
3 Chef
4 Furniture designer/maker
5 Musician
6 Landscape gardener
7 Interior designer
8 Florist
9 Antique dealer
10 Restaurant owner

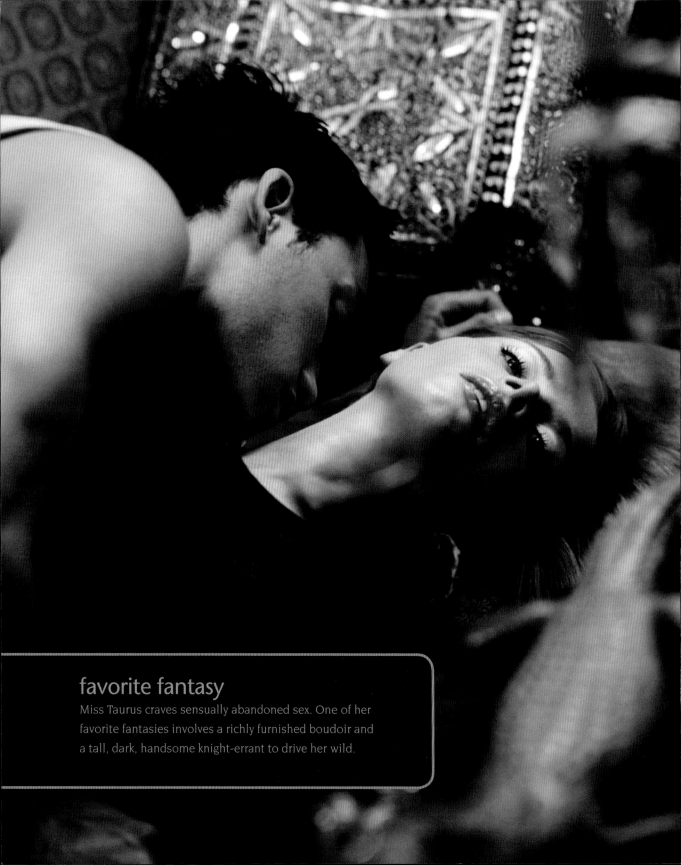

favorite fantasy

Miss Taurus craves sensually abandoned sex. One of her
favorite fantasies involves a richly furnished boudoir and
a tall, dark, handsome knight-errant to drive her wild.

WHAT WORKS FOR HER

Here is one raunchy sign. The Taurus woman's sexuality is strong and deep and thrives on languid, lusty sex. Sensual and romantic, total sexual pleasure is what she gives and what she expects. She makes an amazing lover, as long as you return the favor and treat her like the true love goddess she is.

Tactile sexiness simply oozes out of the lady bull, and she's the diva of voluptuous temptation. In fact, if her earthy appetite isn't satiated with lots of sex, tenderness, and warmth, she'll basically look elsewhere. No "wham bam thank you ma'am" style sex for her: it's all about lengthy foreplay and indulgent closeness. Your five senses are important to her, but what about your sixth? If you can intuitively understand what she's really about and what her sexual needs are, she'll be hooked. One-night stands? If she wants sensual

> She likes lots of sex—and often—so if her partner can't satisfy her, she feels no guilt in looking elsewhere

indulgence, she'll play. But she'd rather wait for Mr. Right and know he's rightfully hers.

A DEMANDING APPETITE

She has an insatiable appetite for sex, plus an erotic fascination with food. She adores sexy feasts:

berries nibbled from her nipples, champagne licked from her clitoris. Sexual locations must be stylishly furnished with silk, satin, lace, and velvets. Let her take the lead when she's in the mood, but secretly she loves to play the submissive partner.

HOW TO MAKE HER HORNY

Most of all, take your time! Miss Taurus thrives on slow, sensual foreplay and is turned on by light kisses and caresses up and down her whole body. Start by paying attention to her face and earlobes, and then gradually make your way down to her sizzling astro-erogenous zone—the throat and neck. Feathery touches around the nape of her

neck and then down to the cleft between her breasts will drive her wild. Follow this up with gentle licks across the top of her shoulders. Now it's time to move in closer. Flicker your lips or eyelashes across her shoulders, dab and dart your tongue over her throat and lips without kissing, and watch her melt with desire. During intercourse, to really get her sizzling, rub the tip of your penis against the ultra-sensitive nape of her neck.

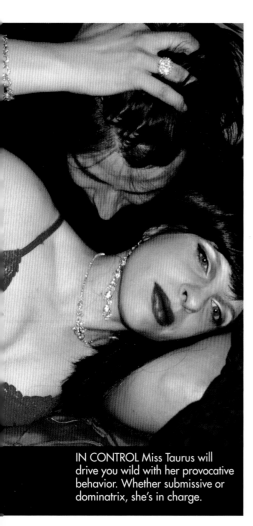

IN CONTROL Miss Taurus will drive you wild with her provocative behavior. Whether submissive or dominatrix, she's in charge.

MISSION: MOST POSSIBLE

The Taurus woman loves erotic foreplay and oral sex: it means she has the emotional closeness and visual contact to maximize her feelings of self-indulgence. But for pure orgasmic bliss, she prefers doggy-style positions and has a fascination for buttocks, just like her male counterpart. For this reason, the Mission Accomplished position is great for satisfying her need for hard, penetrating sex. It stimulates her earthy responsiveness and also ensures she can give ultimate pleasure to you as well, an essential ingredient in her sexual arousal. As an earth sign, Taurus also resonates to the same sexual energy flow as Virgo and Capricorn, so add the Passion Fruit (see pages 112–13) and Orchid positions (see pages 184–85) to her repertoire for a truly orgasmic buzz.

ORAL ANTICS

Remember, this woman hates sex when it's too fast and furious. Quickies won't give her enough time to be fully aroused, and instant penetration without any foreplay means she'll often end up feeling she's missed out. Oral sex allows her to take her time reaching orgasm, and she's also sexually uninhibited when it comes to masturbation. Mutual masturbation gives her incredible libido peaks. She's a secret exhibitionist, and gets turned on by sexy hand-jobs under the restaurant table while you're both sipping fine wines and gourmet feasting. She loves playing a submissive role too, because that domination streak of hers is simply a way of feeling in control. Sneakily, she longs to feel totally out of control so that she can be the rampant earth goddess of carnal delight.

MISSION ACCOMPLISHED

Your Taurus vamp likes to feel totally ravished and this position gives the deep penetration and all-over contact she craves. Let her lie face down on the bed or floor with legs well apart as you kneel between her legs, slowly caressing and kissing her back to stimulate languid, earthy arousal. Ask her to raise her buttocks (a pillow underneath may help) but rest her arms, shoulders, and head on the bed for support.

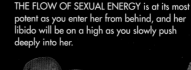
THE FLOW OF SEXUAL ENERGY is at its most potent as you enter her from behind, and her libido will be on a high as you slowly push deeply into her.

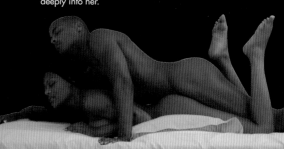

HER TOP TURNOFFS

INFIDELITY
This lady demands total devotion and if she catches you straying, she'll wreak terrible revenge.

LOVE GAMES
She's acutely sensitive. So you'd be advised not to dally with her affections unless you're serious.

LETHARGIC LOVERS
If you can't match her strong sex drive, you'll be thrown out of bed and won't be asked back.

BAD COOKS
If there's one thing she can't stomach, it's a man who doesn't pull his weight in the kitchen.

BAD BREATH
Invest in some mouthwash. Your breath must smell as sweet as this sensual lady does.

DRAMA QUEEN

Once you know her better, bathe together in musky oils while you wash every part of her body for a slow libido buildup, then have oral sex on the floor surrounded by money, jewels, or food. One of Taurus's favorite techniques is to play out her strong sexual fantasies. For a really erotic experience, she might pretend to resist your advances, or reverse the roles and swoop down upon you like a vamp approaching her innocent victim.

Taurus is known to sing sexy songs during lovemaking, or get you horny by whispering dirty stories in your ear. But before you get worried that her mind is wandering from you, remember, it's all an act and just a bit of fun, and deep down she's totally devoted to you. Sex is a deeply emotional act for Taurus, and it's hard for her to have sex and

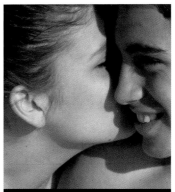

SUGGESTIVE WHISPERS Let her whisper dirty stories and her secret fantasies in your ear and your bull will be at her horniest.

not fall in love. She needs an equally devoted and faithful lover who will treat her like a lady and who can match her powerful appetites for sexual pleasure. This Taurus woman's not looking for bedroom power games, just to enjoy good old-fashioned, natural lust, because that's what makes her feel like the most luscious and sensual of all women that she is.

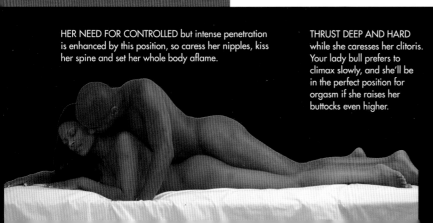

HER NEED FOR CONTROLLED but intense penetration is enhanced by this position, so caress her nipples, kiss her spine and set her whole body aflame.

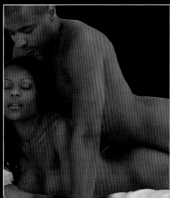

THRUST DEEP AND HARD while she caresses her clitoris. Your lady bull prefers to climax slowly, and she'll be in the perfect position for orgasm if she raises her buttocks even higher.

WHAT WORKS FOR HIM

Not your average bull in a china shop, Mr. Taurus likes to take his time. He's one of the most considerate lovers and aims to please as well as indulge his earthy sex drive. He may not be a three-times-a-night, but one long session with him is enough to confirm he's sex-sational.

Money can buy this man love. With a basic instinct for having the best in life, Taurus is well aware of what's good taste and what isn't, both in and out of bed. When it comes to initial physical contact, he can take forever to make the first move. It's probably best if you do it for him. He also hates aggressive, loud-mouthed women, and is turned on by femininity, grace, and that thing called money. So leave your inner wildcat firmly at home and opt for a classy perfume and a little black dress (feminine-sensual) on that first date, even if you plan on taking it off at the end of the evening.

CREATURE COMFORTS

Taurus gets into the groove very quickly once he knows you're not playing games. But he's got to be in comfortable or beautiful surroundings. Give him a king-size bed or huge floppy sofa, dimmed lights, romantic music, and a little pillow talk about money, beauty, and music, and he's in sexual nirvana. Bulls are very visual. He's ruled by vain Venus, so he's likely to look pretty good himself too, and he's turned on by refined body language and natural, hardly made-up faces. So ditch that tatty G-string and red lipstick and opt for something more subtle and feminine. He adores slinky lingerie, silk panties, and lacy bras—anything that he can get his teeth into and rip off. Literally.

He's a connoisseur of food and sex and wants the finest of both. Sex must be high-caliber sex, it must be worth the effort, and it must taste good. Serve up a gourmet meal followed by sensational sex, and you'll be his gourmet lover forever.

HOW TO MAKE HIM HORNY

Uninhibited about his body, Taurus likes languid and lengthy foreplay whenever he can get it. But do take it slowly. Being an utter sensualist, he's just one big erogenous zone. But for maximum arousal, his astro-zone is focused on the throat. First use a feather or the tips of your fingers and gently trace lines down from the top of his spine to between his buttocks and he'll soon be standing to attention. Next focus on his neck and shoulders. Start behind his earlobes, and with your finger gently stroke him with circular movements. Continue this down to the collarbone and round his throat, then across his shoulders. Next do the same thing using your tongue or lips, tracing lines from the earlobe down the side of his neck, then finishing on the outer edge of his collarbone for sex-tingling arousal.

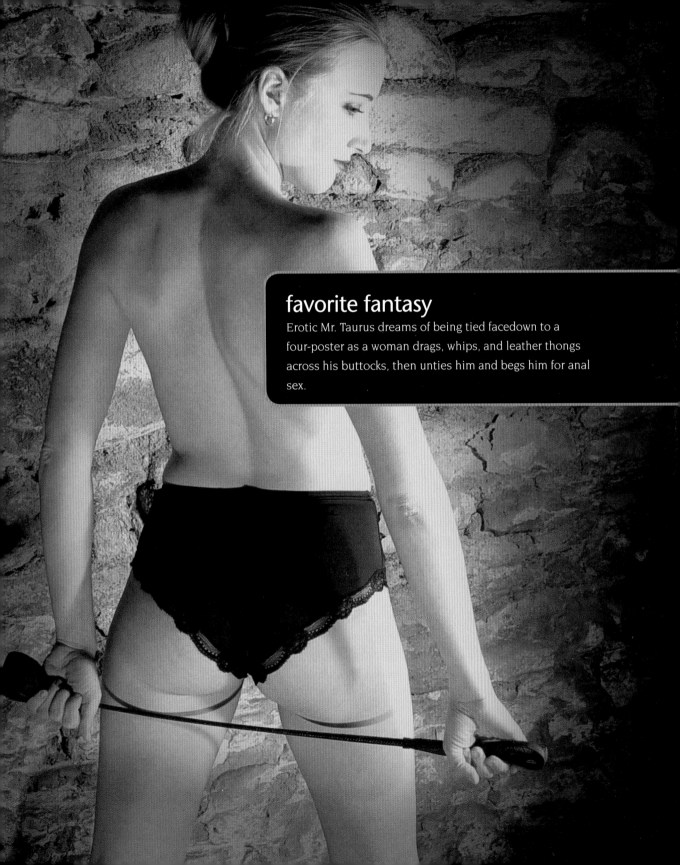

favorite fantasy

Erotic Mr. Taurus dreams of being tied facedown to a four-poster as a woman drags, whips, and leather thongs across his buttocks, then unties him and begs him for anal sex.

PRIMITIVE URGES

Taurus is renowned for his huge sex drive and erection to match. And there really is little to stop him—even if you're begging at the top of your voice! His stamina is truly stunning, and his staying power is his greatest asset. He derives intense stimulation from pleasing you, so the gentlemanly bull is more than willing to make sure that you've hit the big O before satisfying himself.

The only problem with Mr. Taurus is he can be incredibly possessive and jealous. He may not show it on the surface, but flirt with his best mate and you'll be in deepest trouble. He believes that his possessions are his and his alone, and that includes you. And if you're happy to be under his control, his emotional and sexual mastery makes for explosively pleasurable bedroom antics.

ORALLY YOURS

He adores oral sex in sensual, lush surroundings: on a velvet sofa or a four-poster bed draped in fake furs. He loves the feel of lace, leather, and food against his skin. Gently tie him to your bedposts and smother his belly and penis with champagne, yogurt, or honey. Lick it off slowly and seductively. Ask him to eat cherries or strawberries from between your breasts. And suck his fingers while he nibbles your nipples. Go for long, lazy afternoons having sex in the country or by the sea. Anywhere he can get back to nature. Have sex in long grass and tickle his belly with flowers or feathers. He's turned on by playing a submissive role too, so sit astride him and then bring yourself to orgasm while he watches you. Pretend that you're an aromatherapist

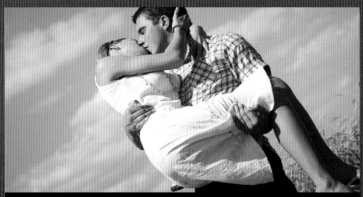

BACK TO NATURE Go picnicking in the park or countryside and earthy Mr. Taurus will be up for sex in the open air.

MAN ON A MISSION

Mr. Taurus loves basic, straightforward sex. The Missionary position is a great way to maintain his stamina and staying power, and means he can vary his position and yours very easily without breaking up the intense physical and emotional closeness. Alternatively, when he's in one of his lazy-bull, submissive moods, try sitting on top of him so he can watch himself entering you for maximum arousal.

MISSIONARY STYLE ALLOWS close-up eye contact, making him feel adored and emotionally secure. Don't forget that, for all his macho image, he's got a vulnerable side too.

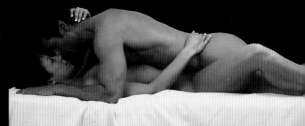

and massage his buttocks. He's often up for anal sex too, but if you're not, lean forward against a tree when you're on that country ramble, let him take you from behind, and tell him to fantasize about it instead. Ask him to lick your

waters by stroking the perineum (the smooth bit between the testicles and the anus) using two or three fingers. Massage quite firmly. Let your fingers casually brush against his anus and see how he reacts. If he pulls away or clenches his

The **benevolent bull** has strong **passions** and **large appetites**—in every sense

fingers while you masturbate yourself with them. Then give him a blowjob while he slides his fingers deep inside you.

THE BOTTOM LINE

Your Taurus man is fascinated by buttocks. In fact, he's a bit of a bottom-watcher. (And that includes both sexes.) Test the

buttocks, then don't insist! If he seems keen, gently explore further. If he's not up for anal entry (because not all Taurean men are), he'll adore it if you rub your breasts against his buttocks, kiss him in the cleft of his buttocks and around his testicles, then tongue the outside of his anus.

HIS TOP TURNOFFS

UGLINESS
Never let him catch you shaving your armpits or wearing a face-mask. He simply can't bear to think of you as anything less than a goddess.

PLAYING HARD TO GET
The more you play games, the more enraged he'll get. Just be straight with him and he will be straight with you.

POVERTY
Never say you're broke. He's terrified of financial insecurity and would sell his soul rather than live with a penniless woman.

STUBBORNNESS
Don't lock horns with him because he's just not going to give way. There's not enough room in a relationship for two bulls.

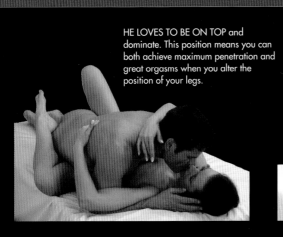

HE LOVES TO BE ON TOP and dominate. This position means you can both achieve maximum penetration and great orgasms when you alter the position of your legs.

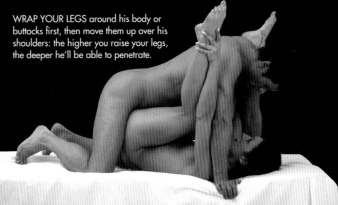

WRAP YOUR LEGS around his body or buttocks first, then move them up over his shoulders: the higher you raise your legs, the deeper he'll be able to penetrate.

IS THIS THE ONE?

Taureans need someone who takes great pleasure in the simple things of life and will always be there for them. So if you want commitment, security, and indulgence, you might be the perfect match for the sexually insatiable bull.

ARIES AND TAURUS

Aries is always on the go, while Taurus would rather flop around at home. But you are fascinated by your differences. You'll share anything from a sauna to a bunk bed, but watch out that Taurus doesn't fall asleep just when Aries is ready for more.

TAURUS AND TAURUS

Likely to be spending most of your time on the horizontal! Lots of silent tenacity and mutual defiance out of the bedroom, but a wonderful earthy rapport as long as you both communicate. Security-conscious, you're cool with money too.

GEMINI AND TAURUS

Taurus gets possessive; Gemini hates being possessed. Great for a short-lived romance, but Gemini's unreliable streak angers Taurus and Gemini soon gets tired of the bull's obsession with self-indulgence.

CANCER AND TAURUS

Together you'll create an easy-going lifestyle, because neither is into points scoring. Cancer loves those cozy nights in tasting Taurus's gourmet skills. Taurus adores the close rapport. Sexually, the bedsheets will be sizzling

LEO AND TAURUS

Taurus is cautious and languid; Leo is flamboyant and wants fire-and-brimstone sex. You're both stubborn and self-centered, so the sparks will fly. Rarely long-lasting, but sexually exciting and hypnotic.

VIRGO AND TAURUS

A warm, trusting rapport and superb workable relationship, long-lasting and stable. Once you realize that you have a joint love of nature, as well as a sensual and sexy rapport, there's very little to keep you apart.

Both ruled by sexy Venus, you're "oh so vain," and will out-flirt each other at any social event. But Libra's perfectionist streak will eventually drive Taurus up the wall. And once the romance has worn off, Libra finds Taurus far too possessive.

LIBRA AND TAURUS

Either a highly explosive relationship or intense and permanent. One of the most potent and arousing sexual clashes in the zodiac. Scorpio is fascinated by Taurus's earthy sexuality, and Taurus by Scorpio's extremes of passion.

SCORPIO AND TAURUS

Strangely, can be quite satisfying, as long as Taurus doesn't get too possessive. This is a long-term rapport that can gain strength. Sagittarius, however, likes to roam, Taurus to stay put. Sexually compelling.

SAGITTARIUS AND TAURUS

Physically and mentally in tune, but you could end up in fights about who controls the finances. A great match for long-term commitment. You both want to be a successful couple in the eyes of the world, and often make it to the top together.

CAPRICORN AND TAURUS

Very different perception of life and unlikely to get beyond a few shags. Aquarius is unconventional and not as interested in the emotional or physical aspects of love as conservative Taurus. You won't find much to get off on, in or out of bed.

AQUARIUS AND TAURUS

Good romantic rapport, as Pisces feels safe in reliable hands. But Taurus can get confused by Pisces' dream world and sensitive nature. Sexually, the fish can drop all inhibitions, cradled by the bull's down-to-earth approach to love.

PISCES AND TAURUS

AND THE WINNER IS...

For long-term commitment, Taurus can find a good mental and emotional affinity with Virgo and Capricorn. For sexual closeness and home comforts, warm-hearted Cancer gets high marks.

And for scorching sex and passion, a sizzling liaison with Scorpio is not to be missed. But if there has to be an outright winner, it's Capricorn. These two earth signs both want a relationship based on long-term commitment, where they feel financially and emotionally secure.

LONG-TERM LOVE WITH TAURUS

The good news is Taurus is one sign of the zodiac who, once committed, will be yours for life. The bad news is, this fixed earth sign is ferociously stubborn and equally possessive. So never tussle with a Taurus, or you'll find yourself at the center of a bullfight you can't win. But with dedication and understanding of their psyche, Taureans make the most generous and supportive of long-term partners.

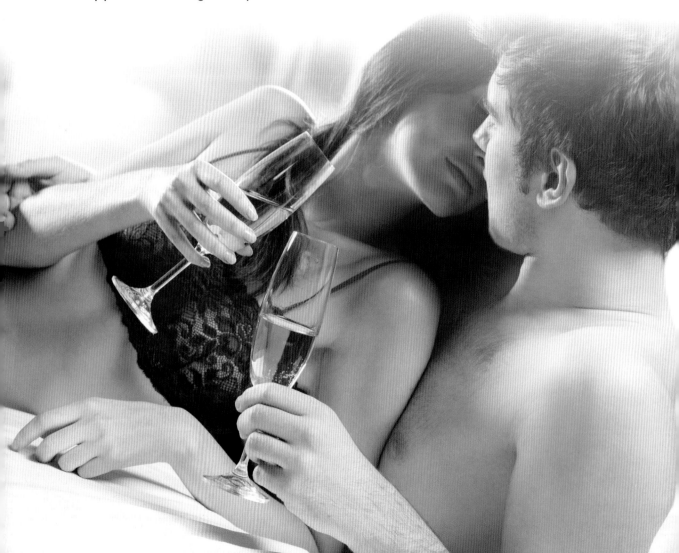

If you can match Taurus blow for blow in the bedroom, there's great hope for your joint future. To keep hold of your bull, you have to be as sexually indulgent as he or she is. But it's not just endurance: Taurus thrives on five-star sex and emotional closeness. So if you've harbored secret fantasies of threesomes, or still have your ex-lovers dropping by for coffee (or drinks), then forget the bull now. But if you're looking for a considerate,

financially secure homelife. Help out with all those DIY projects, spend evenings in front of the log fire, and you'll be rewarded with a steadfast, loving, and affectionate partner.

NEST EGG
The way to the Taurean heart is truly through the stomach! If you're not a great chef, join your bull in the kitchen, and follow Taurus's instructions to the letter. Showing faith in their culinary

MAKE YOUR BULL SEE RED

If there's one thing a bull won't tolerate, it's cheating. Taureans put great emphasis on monogamous relationships. If they suspect their security is being threatened or feel in danger of being exploited, they'll be off. So if you want the bull to dump you, the trick is to leave tell-tale signs of infidelity like lipstick on your collar or mysterious cufflinks under the pillow. The whiff of a stranger's perfume or aftershave on the pillow is the kind of metaphorical red rag that makes a bull charge right out of your life.

> If you supply **masses** of adoring **attention** and say **"I love you"** at any time of day, your bull will be **hooked** for life

consistent lover to grow old with, then Taurus is the one for you.

HOME COMFORTS
Bulls need constant reassurance that you love them more than anyone else in the world. If you can accept their possessiveness, and realize this is a result of a deep-seated fear of rejection, then they will do anything for you. So make sure you're equally committed to a comfortable and

skills implies you have utter faith and trust in them too. Be enthusiastic about planning long-term joint projects, but let Taurus run the finances—if your bull feels in charge of the purse-strings, he or she won't charge anywhere except to your side. Above all, Taurus is a loyal lover who will stick with you through thick and thin as long as you support the bull's need for a secure and consistent lifestyle.

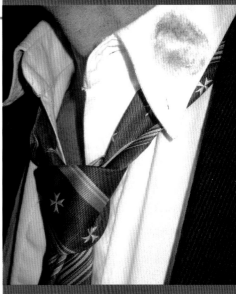

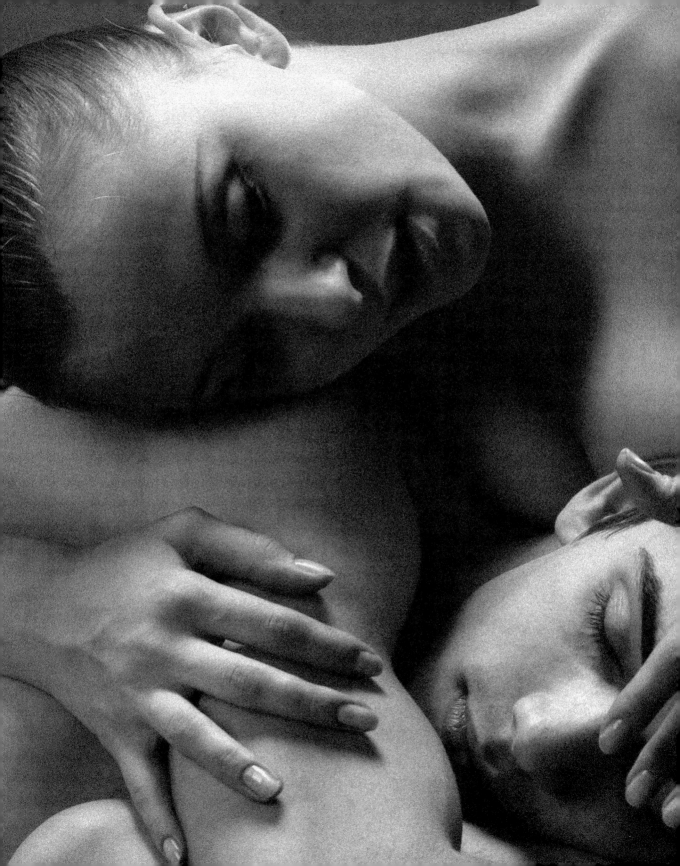

GEMINI

MAY 22 — JUNE 21

STAR STATS

Ruling planet MERCURY
Signature symbol THE TWINS
Metal QUICKSILVER
Stone AGATE
Color YELLOW

Where to find Gemini Bookshops, Internet cafés, mobile phone shops, or working in the media.

Hot date Take Gemini to a carnival or a party; they just love to play!

Needs and desires Witty and light-hearted, Gemini needs communication by the bucketful, both in and out of bed.

Top turn-on Erotic conversations over the phone.

Sex positions ♀ Genie Rub
♂ On a Role

Sex toy A set of love eggs, to arouse curiosity and libido simultaneously.

Sex statistic 90 percent of Geminis think about someone other than their partner while having sex.

WHAT TO EXPECT WITH GEMINI

Changeable, restless, and unpredictable, Geminis are as curious about love as they are about the world. The sign of the twins is about duality. So always remember that when you fall for a Gemini, you're getting two people for the price of one. Endlessly entertaining, this air sign can also be double trouble!

Gemini is without doubt the most amusing and romantic of the air signs, but also the most frustrating. Ruled by Mercury, the messenger of the gods, your double package of fun is also elusive and terrified of losing personal freedom. Yet Geminis love falling in love: they adore the romance and playing games, fooling around, bluffing, changing their minds, and generally making you feel as if you really aren't exactly sure who they are and what they're up to. Geminis will tell the odd little white lie, both to tease and also to just test themselves against you.

CHARMING FLIRTS
It's their bubbly charm and witty replies that make Geminis renowned as the biggest flirts in the zodiac. They'll pretend they're fascinated by your every word, and then suddenly go off on a tangent and chat up your best friend. Male or female, Geminis are independent and light-hearted. They hate routine and conventional assumptions about love relationships. The twins are far more interested in the quality of your mind than your sexual performance. If you can stimulate their brains first, bodies second, then you'll be in with a chance to get more intimate with these romantic, intellectual magicians.

CAPRICIOUS
What can be done about the changeable, airy Gemini nature? Not a lot. Accept that they can be fickle, footloose, and have a pretty neurotic sex drive. But if they do fall in love, they'll be devoted, as long as you're willing to spend nights solving crossword puzzles, and change sex positions and habits often. For the charmer of the zodiac, love and sex are entertainment.

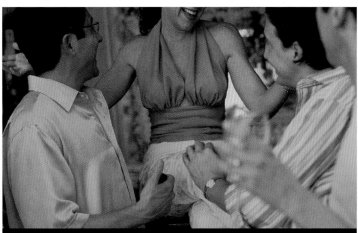

SPOILED FOR CHOICE Fun-loving and gregarious, Gemini just can't resist any opportunity to play the outrageous flirt.

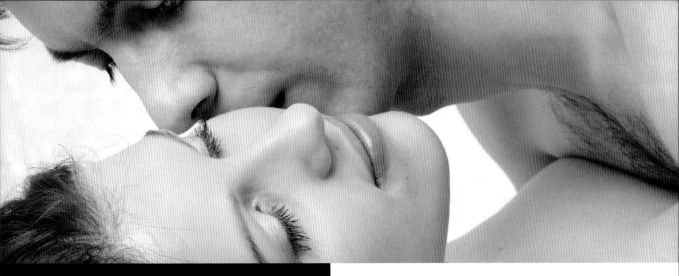

THE GEMINI MAN

This is one difficult man to understand. Laid-back and youthful, he doesn't exactly ooze masculinity or advertise that he's a walking sex bomb. Yet behind the charm and clever words, the Gemini

If you're the **jealous** or **possessive** type, then **stay away**

man has a restless and opportunist sex drive. He's a game-player looking for a woman who can match him for objectivity, romance, and brainpower. Mr. Popular is surrounded by fascinated females, but he's seduced by unpredictable women who can laugh at all his gags and crack their own.

THE GEMINI WOMAN

Intelligent and witty, she's usually the center of social attention. In fact, her entourage of adoring male friends could irritate you—unless you become one too. Vibrant and energetic, she falls for independent men, travelers, and intellectual gurus. But Gemini is essentially lonely. Always searching for that elusive "twin," there's something quite soulful about her behind the charades and the restless, ever-changing personality. She mirrors herself in those around her, and often moves from lover to lover in the hope that someone will satisfy her inner needs and erotic sexuality. Her light and breezy approach to sex is all too frequently misunderstood by men, and she often gives too easily of her body because she assumes that this is the key to being loved and finding a soul mate. Ironically, what she needs to discover is that the missing twin is within herself.

GEMINI IN A NUTSHELL

KEYWORDS Mercurial; entertaining; talkative; witty; inconsistent; freedom-loving; game-playing; charming
LIKES Variety; discussing every subject under the sun; erotic phone conversations; being unpredictable in bed
DISLIKES Know-it-alls; possessiveness; a routine lifestyle

TRACKING DOWN YOUR GEMINI

They're elusive and inconsistent, so you're not going to find it easy to catch yourself a Gemini. But if you're as flighty as the twins are, you may well bump into them on your travels. Extrovert Geminis have a habit of chatting to anyone they meet in airports, bars, and social venues.

Restless Geminis adore flitting here, there, and everywhere. One minute they're off on a fast-paced shopping trip, the next they're painting their kitchens, then they're off to the local bar

OPPORTUNITY KNOCKS

Gemini seeks an active and dramatic lifestyle. With a talent for taking on more than one project at a time, the twins can be infuriatingly unreliable too.

This is one **sociable** sign, so check out where the **crowds** are **forming** and there might be a Gemini **at the center**

to gossip and be entertained. Keeping up with them isn't going to be easy, unless you're willing to hang on to their shirt tails or be as gregarious and outgoing as they are. Because they are born communicators, you're most likely to find them working in the media, but with their love of travel, they also make great taxi drivers, tour operators, and airport staff.

When they say they'll meet you next week, make sure you call to remind them. They have short attention spans and can often forget your name after they've just met you! You're likely to find them on bar stools chatting the night away, or signing up for a new course of study. However, the chances are they won't be in the same place you left them. So if you pop out to the restroom,

Gemini may have met someone far more fascinating by the time you return. And if you sign up for that course just to get to know the twins better, chances are they'll have given up after the first lesson.

GOOD COMMUNICATOR

Geminis usually work in an environment where they can feed information or create clever ideas and punchy messages. Advertising, sales, and journalism all suit their mercurial minds. The Roman god Mercury, their mythical ruler, was able to visit heaven, the earth, and the underworld, bringing novel ideas and fascinating tales to those who were stuck on only one level of existence. Geminis are his true heirs and love flexing their versatile minds, communicating new ideas, or explaining how to get from point A to point B. in the shortest possible time.

PLACES TO LOOK

INTERNET CAFÉ/LIBRARY

Geminis's curiosity is never satisfied, and they're forever on the Internet researching their latest craze or nosing around in all those musty old books for clues and answers to some of life's perplexing questions.

LOCAL BAR

Geminis do have a habit of popping into and out of the local bar on a regular basis. They just want to entertain as many different people as possible. But be warned that they can also disappear at a moment's notice.

PARTIES

Geminis usually linger near the drinks table to await the inevitable adoring throng. Include yourself in this heaving mass of would-be seducers but, to outsmart the competition, be provocative.

GEMINI TOP TEN CAREERS

1	Journalist	6	Writer
2	Bookseller	7	Telephone sales person
3	Advertising executive	8	Taxi driver
4	Courier	9	Illustrator
5	Linguist	10	Newsreader/Narrator

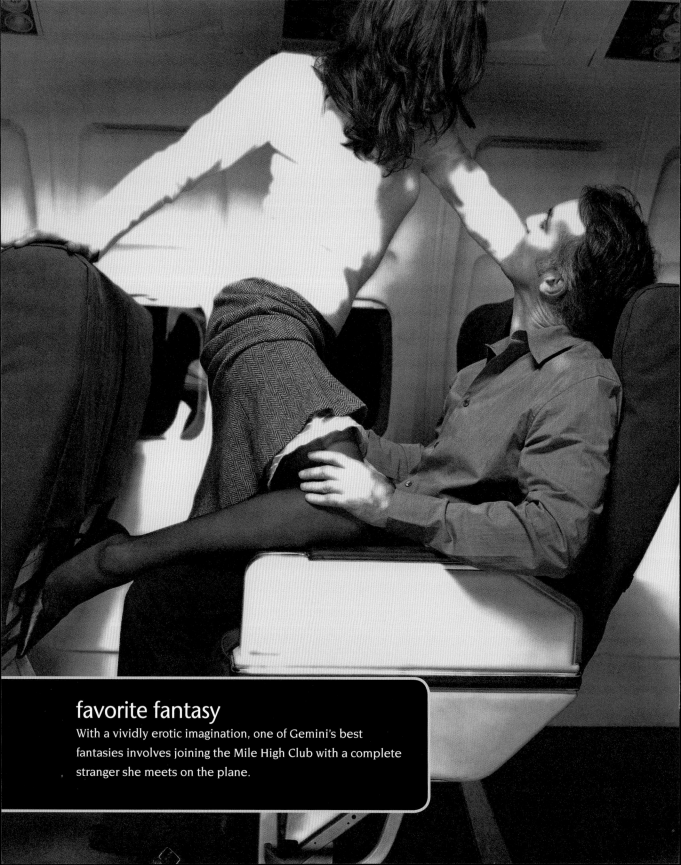

favorite fantasy

With a vividly erotic imagination, one of Gemini's best fantasies involves joining the Mile High Club with a complete stranger she meets on the plane.

WHAT WORKS FOR HER

The Gemini woman's sexuality is erratic. There are times when she thinks about sex 24/7, and others when she's more interested in discussing the latest space-shuttle launch. But if you're as freedom-loving, intelligent, and unpredictable as she is, then she'll amuse you not only in bed but out of it as well.

Variety is the spice of a Gemini's love life. She's a romantic, falls in love instantly with a face, mind, or voice, and often jumps into bed too fast without thinking about why she's there. It's not that she's promiscuous, but she can be rather naive about other people's intentions, and is often let down by one-night wonders or men who think she's a flirt with no desire for commitment. Secretly, she wants a permanent lover by her side, but she needs her freedom too.

She thrives on a variety of sensations, and she has a more

> Never just think that **she's the one** with Gemini—this twin soul is **double the fun!**

intellectual approach to sex than most other signs. She likes to "think" about sex, and often prefers fantasizing during oral sex to long-haul penetration.

TWO FOR ONE

She may seem emotionally uninvolved but that's just a cover-up for her fear of her own feelings. Her expectations are so high that she finds it difficult to separate love and sex. If you're looking for a one-night stand and think this woman's lighthearted and promiscuous, take care. Remember, you're getting two women for the price of one: the outgoing entertainer and the vulnerable child.

HOW TO MAKE HER HORNY

Talk to her. Gemini's astro-erogenous zone is her brain. She's not a touchy-feely type of woman but is erotically stimulated by words, thoughts, and the power of her mind. It can take Gemini a long time to be aroused via normal foreplay, but if you talk

do. Kiss her hands and suck her fingers gently, then lick the inside of her arms, all sensitive erogenous zones for the Mercurial woman. At this point, she'll probably say that she wants to take over, because Geminis like to "get on with it." Don't be too slow and sensual or she'll only get bored: the more teasing and unpredictable you are with your

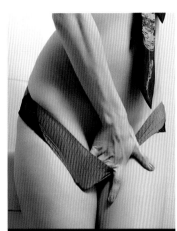

HANDS DOWN, THE WINNER! Spontaneous masturbation is her favorite turn-on, and she'll love showing you how it's done.

SPONTANEOUS

The Gemini woman is not into heavy panting all-night sessions, and she'd rather have sex when she feels like it, spontaneous and uninhibited. But she does need to play, and that means lots of seductive gestures, wicked comments, and giggling sexual antics. You must be able to communicate your sexiest secrets, be capable of having sex while talking about it, or phoning your friends while she's masturbating you, then spend the rest of the day on your mobile making saucy suggestions about what you're going to do later.

TWICE AS NICE

She has a natural ability for multiple orgasms and isn't afraid to show off her favorite masturbation techniques. Flirty Gemini loves fantasizing that you're strangers who've just met. She never feels guilty about having sex, even when she knows she's with someone she shouldn't be (and that can be an arousal factor). However, she may well regret her spontaneous sex drive if she finds you were only after a one-night stand.

Gemini can blow away the cobwebs from your inhibitions, too (if you have any). Remember, she has such an erotic mind that she can bring herself to orgasm without either of you touching. She's not particularly turned on by sweaty sensual indulgence. In fact, Gemini gets turned on by the whole prelude to sex rather than the act itself. She's a mean hand with a dildo, and if you're as versatile and experimental as she is, then pretty much anything goes.

VISUAL AIDS

Visual and aural stimulation also gets her libido going. Mobile phones were invented for Gemini, so ask her to call you in the office while she's masturbating, or vice versa! Or phone each other from the same bed, and ask her to do exactly what you tell her, while you watch. Place a mirror in front of the bed and let her watch as you give her oral sex. Read erotic literature or watch

GENIE RUB

The Genie Rub position will enable your Gemini to get maximum enjoyment through an ever-changing variety of sexual contact. If you can roll over without withdrawing your penis, then you'll both experience pure sex in motion! Changing angle with you still inside her ensures her arousal level can peak while you're in transition. To start, lie on your sides face-to-face, so she has visual and verbal contact.

SLIDE YOUR BODY between her legs, until you can feel your penis against her vulva. As she twines her ankles around your legs, move rhythmically together.

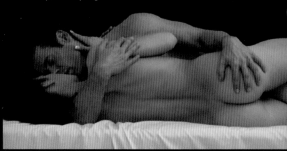

HER TOP TURNOFFS

CHAUVINISTS

She needs a man who respects her as an intellectual equal or you won't stay long in her company.

GETTING TOO PHYSICAL

She's interested in romantic, erotic intimacy, not the nuts and bolts of heavy breathing, sweaty backs, and men obsessed with the size of their penises.

POSSESSIVENESS

Gemini can't bear a man who thinks he owns her. She values her freedom and if you start wondering where she is or what she's doing, you'll be left wondering forever.

BOREDOM

Change your techniques, follow her lead, and be as inspirational in bed as she is. The same old routine equals stagnant and boring loving.

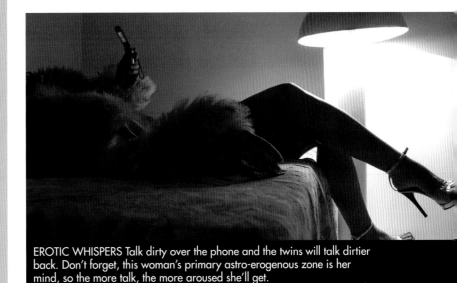

EROTIC WHISPERS Talk dirty over the phone and the twins will talk dirtier back. Don't forget, this woman's primary astro-erogenous zone is her mind, so the more talk, the more aroused she'll get.

a dirty video together while you take her from behind.

Gemini loves to dominate and prefers a multitude of sex positions to just one standard. However, she adores the Genie Rub position because it can lead on to a variety of other experimental and visually stimulating positions. What Gemini doesn't want is long penetrative thrusting without a change of position. In fact, she's determined to show you that she has an extraordinary repertoire of sexual skills, and masturbating herself is often preferable to waiting for a lover who cannot respond to her speedy arousal.

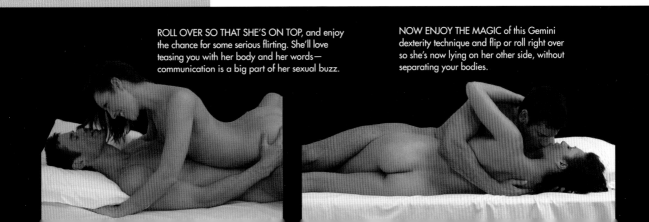

ROLL OVER SO THAT SHE'S ON TOP, and enjoy the chance for some serious flirting. She'll love teasing you with her body and her words—communication is a big part of her sexual buzz.

NOW ENJOY THE MAGIC of this Gemini dexterity technique and flip or roll right over so she's now lying on her other side, without separating your bodies.

WHAT WORKS FOR HIM

The archetypal charmer of the zodiac, you never know quite where you are with the Mr. Gemini. And that includes in bed as well as out of it. He's perfected the art of role playing different sexual characters, not to gain power over you, but, well, just to have fun.

A bit of a will-o'-the-wisp, your Gemini man is often more turned on by the idea of sex than by the actual performance. But if you're up for tangled sheets, spontaneous romping, and laughter, this man is the most lighthearted and versatile lover around. Mr. Gemini is chatty and loves sexy phone calls. On a first date, don't be surprised if he's on the phone more than he's on to you. And any hint of jealousy, and he might well perform one of his famous Houdini disappearing acts in front of your very eyes. But if you can chatter about anything under the sun and put up with his instant fascination with every woman that walks into the bar, then he'll feel secure that you're not just interested in his body but his brain as well.

PETER PAN CHARM

Youthful, erratic, and downright cheeky, he often seems more like a child than a man. Behind that witty facade, he's actually a true romantic, but he hates revealing his emotions and insecurities or talking about sloppy aspects of love. Deep involvement isn't easy for him, which is why he has a reputation for being a tad promiscuous. He is excited by the short term, the now, the latest angle of light on your face, the bead of sweat running between your breasts. He can also be quite devious about his sexual needs too. If he's in your bed or dragged you into an alley on the first date, then beware: he might also be out of the bed or back in that restaurant chatting up someone new before you know it. Keep him on his toes by showing that you're as flirtatious, freedom loving, and independent as he is.

HOW TO MAKE HIM HORNY

Have an erotic conversation across the restaurant table or in the back seat of the taxi, to get him going. The more suggestive you are, the more he'll be tuned into his primary astro-erogenous zone, his brain. Bodily arousal isn't difficult for Mr. Gemini; it's just not the best way to raise his libido level. So forget about sensual soppiness. What will make him horny is spontaneous foreplay, and lots of saucy chat while you're doing it. Stand face-to-face but still dressed and kiss his neck and face while you run your fingers under his shirt and down to his belly. Tell him what you're going to do to him each step of the way as you move your hand down to his penis. He adores quick moves, so don't hang around doing one thing for long. Then make it clear you're up for oral sex, now!

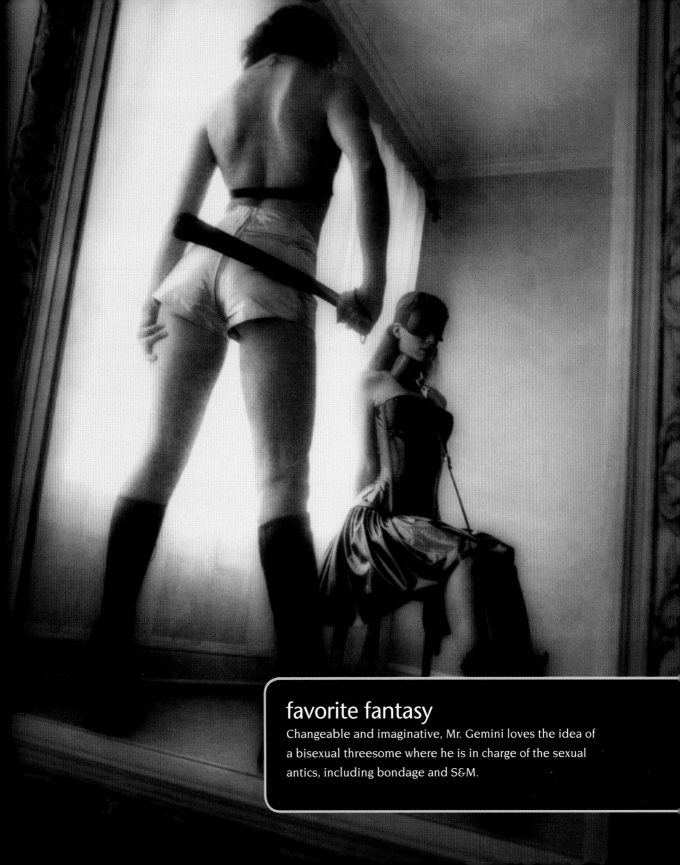

favorite fantasy

Changeable and imaginative, Mr. Gemini loves the idea of
a bisexual threesome where he is in charge of the sexual
antics, including bondage and S&M.

FUN-LOVING

Mr. Gemini likes to flex his mind. And when it comes to talking, then sex is one of his favorite topics. How do women manage to have multiple orgasms? What's the latest scientific view about the sex lives of apes? You name it, he'll know about it. But when it comes to grand passion, torrid feelings, and burning desire, then you have to look elsewhere. This man thrives on entertainment and sexual variety. He's easily seduced with words and roleplay. "Let's pretend…" was invented for Gemini.

UNPREDICTABLE

The Gemini man likes the thrill of quick arousal rather than lengthy sex sessions. He'll clown around, but you never know quite where you stand. Is he plotting how to get your panties off, or how to leave in the morning before he gets horny? He's not trying to avoid sex—it's his favorite pastime—but he can't stand being ruled by his sex drive. Mr. Gemini is unpredictable, but he's great fun and doesn't pretend to be a walking sex bomb.

GAME, SET, AND MATCH

Play nude snakes and ladders, strip poker, or other board games. Laughter turns him on, so the funnier oral sex is, the better his orgasm. Make love on bubble wrap, or on a chair. Anywhere that isn't the bed! Tell him over a candlelit dinner that you're not wearing any panties, and you're going to perform a striptease for him. Then do it in a public place, discreetly of course.

Masturbate him in a public place, like the subway, the top of the stairs at a party, or even on a bridge at dusk. Tell him to fantasize that you're a stranger he's just met on a train, and then he'll play the kind of games you choose, especially if they involve sexual forfeits. Play tic-tac-toe, and the first time you lose bend over, pull your panties to one side, and have sex on the table. Read him an

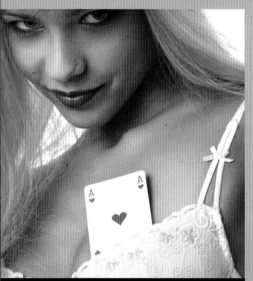

GAME-PLAYER The Gemini man gets off on sexy card games, especially ones where you hold all the aces.

ON A ROLE

Gemini prefers equality of position, where you can both move quickly and easily and change positions when the mood takes him, which is frequently! Sexual intimacy has to be about playing different roles for the Gemini man to feel secure enough to orgasm. This sequence will hold his interest as each position allows him to play a new role, with plenty of opportunites for mutual mastubation and dirty talk.

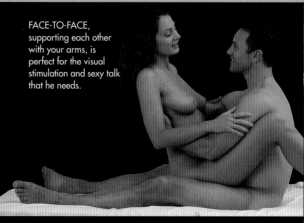

FACE-TO-FACE, supporting each other with your arms, is perfect for the visual stimulation and sexy talk that he needs.

erotic novel, while he rubs his penis all over your body for the ultimate mutual buzz.

ELUSIVE

Now you see him, now you don't. Well, to be honest, he is a little devious, and can flirt with your

INTER ALIA

Gemini's mastery of erotic turn-ons and oral stimulation is unrivaled. However, penetrative sex and lengthy thrusting can be a big issue for him. Orgasm makes him feel vulnerable, and the dynamics of repetitive sex

> Be prepared for **change** and **novelty** with Gemini, or he'll decide **three's a crowd**

best friend or talk about sex to other women in fun, but it's only because he loves to play with ideas and words. Although he can be a bit of a slippery customer, if you can keep him constantly on a mental high and never appear to be jealous, Mr. Gemini will be your sexiest ever companion and lover.

become dull. He's most likely to enjoy climaxing in your mouth or across your breasts to add variety and spice to intercourse. Ask a Gemini man for sexual stimulation and he'll give it with variety and unsurpassed know-how. But try to make him stick to one routine and he'll put on those Mercurial wings and fly.

HIS TOP TURNOFFS

JEALOUSY

This is one independent and freedom-loving man, so make sure you never show your green eyes when he's chatting up your best friend or he'll just disappear in a puff of (green) smoke.

EMOTIONAL STUFF

If you don't have a sense of humor and proportion about life and love, then get out now. Mr. Gemini really can't bear weepy women, and he detests emotional outpourings.

MARRIAGE

It's not that he doesn't want a lover or friend, but he hates looking as if he's attached to any one person. He's hardly marriage material, so don't mention aisles, vows, or rings or he'll run rings round you.

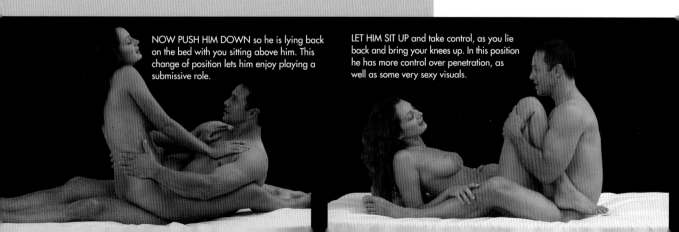

NOW PUSH HIM DOWN so he is lying back on the bed with you sitting above him. This change of position lets him enjoy playing a submissive role.

LET HIM SIT UP and take control, as you lie back and bring your knees up. In this position he has more control over penetration, as well as some very sexy visuals.

IS THIS THE ONE?

Gemini is a sign that values freedom more than commitment. But if you can take a philosophical perspective on love and life and enjoy changing scenery and friends as much as the twins do, they might just stick around.

ARIES AND GEMINI

Great physical rapport here, and sexually both are adventurous. Only problem is Aries is too self-centered and pushy, and can't match Gemini for mind games. Fun-loving, spirited, but eventually exhausting.

TAURUS AND GEMINI

Taurus loves routine, Gemini anything but! Fascinated by each other's different sexual needs, but ultimately Taurus can't keep up with the madcap and unpredictable side of the twins, and Gemini quickly gets bored of all that eating.

GEMINI AND GEMINI

Identical twins. Intellectually stimulating and always buzzing with new ideas both in and out of bed. Good for roaming about like a couple of kids, but you're both led astray by a beautiful face, so chances of stability are virtually zero.

CANCER AND GEMINI

Cancer makes Gemini feel quite like settling down. For a while anyway. But Gemini soon tires of Cancer's clinginess and Cancer of Gemini's flighty flirtatious streak. Physically compelling but hard to sustain.

LEO AND GEMINI

Gemini lives in the head, but Leo lives in the heart. Although Leos adore the twins' witty charm, they can't be sure of complete loyalty. Leo wants to be treated like royalty, and Gemini likes flirting with the entourage. Not an easy match.

VIRGO AND GEMINI

Instant attraction or repulsion. Intellectually, Virgos think they're brighter than Geminis and criticize every move they make. Could be fun for a quick fling, but is lacking long-term affinity.

Immediate rapport as you both have sexy, hilarious minds. Neither want emotional intensity and your adaptability keeps each other on your toes. Great for fun and romantic sex if Geminis are kept amused and Libras aren't put-upon.

Very different natures at work and an interesting erotic connection. Can be a complete love-hate affair. Sexually wild and unpredictable, but Scorpio's too jealous and Gemini's too fickle for long-term loving.

Natural opposites in the zodiac, so sure to be fireworks. A magnetic sexual attraction, and usually fast paced and furious. Exciting and adventurous, and you'll both accept the freedom factor of the other.

Gemini is bound to be curious about how the goat ticks. But that's about as far as it will go. Capricorns are too conventional and stuck in their ways and will want to control Geminis' fickleness. Sexually difficult.

Excellent intellectual rapport: an inspiring, unpredictable relationship. But Aquarius spends hours analyzing Gemini, while the twins would rather be out and about. Good sexual affinity, and possibly long-lasting if both stay independent.

Both unpredictable and changeable, Pisces will be easily led astray by Gemini's charm. Sexually fascinated by each other, but you could both be so elusive that you never really get that close.

AND THE WINNER IS...

Trap a butterfly and it doesn't live very long. And Geminis do like to flit from partner to partner, or at least have the space to lead their free-spirited lifestyles. For a fling or brief affair, Aries, Pisces, and Virgo could get them excited for a while. But for long-term rapport the two other air signs, Aquarius and Libra, come up trumps. On the other hand, for sexual dynamite, romance, and adventure, Gemini's life will turn upside-down for the better with a Sagittarian.

LONG-TERM LOVE WITH GEMINI

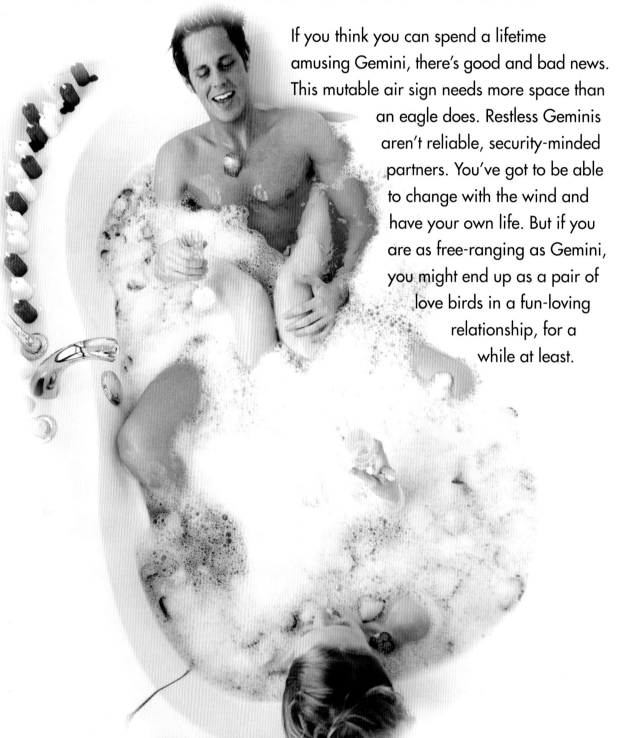

If you think you can spend a lifetime amusing Gemini, there's good and bad news. This mutable air sign needs more space than an eagle does. Restless Geminis aren't reliable, security-minded partners. You've got to be able to change with the wind and have your own life. But if you are as free-ranging as Gemini, you might end up as a pair of love birds in a fun-loving relationship, for a while at least.

Never assume you're going to become a loved-up couple just because Gemini falls for you. The trickster of the zodiac often believes "this is it," but the chances are that a few weeks or months into the relationship, your mercurial lover will be talking about his or her latest plans for the future, which may not include you. If Geminis ever do use the word "we," it's most likely that they're referring to their double selves. But join in their lighthearted banter, and they might come to believe you're part of the equation too.

BRIGHT AND BREEZY

Geminis can't stand dull people or situations, so you're going to have to play the part of a party animal. Throw yourself heart and soul into social occasions. Indulge the Gemini desire for flirting, chitchat, and witty interaction with all other members of the opposite sex, and agree that "so-and-so is very attractive" and "such-and-such has an amazing brain." Above all, make sure you get out there and have your own fun too. Rather than try to tame the twins, be as spontaneous and changeable as they are, and they won't get bored.

SEX IN THE CITY

The twins like to think they're not tied down or committed to anyone, simply because they fear the responsibility of it all. So be flexible, and create the illusion of freedom. Be open to moving house or country every six months (or at least moving the furniture around); enjoy the city but show that you're happy to get out of town on impulse; and be wild and impulsive about life generally. If you learn to relax and embrace change, Gemini will give you a fresh perspective on life and how exciting it can be.

LOSING THE TWINS

The surest way to get mercurial Geminis to fly from your side is to bore them. Tell them very long jokes with weak punch lines, or discuss the state of the economy for at least an hour. Alternatively, watch the television night after night and don't talk to them. Lack of communication is the kiss of death to Gemini. Once you've seen them yawn more than once, there'll be no more kisses of any kind—not even a good-bye one as they head off in search of someone far more fascinating.

> This could be a **fun-filled** and **exhilarating** partnership, as long as you can cope with Gemini's **short attention span**

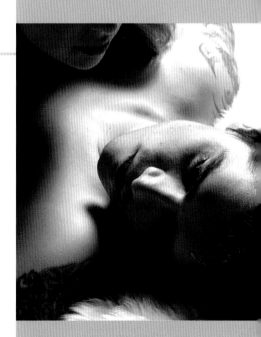

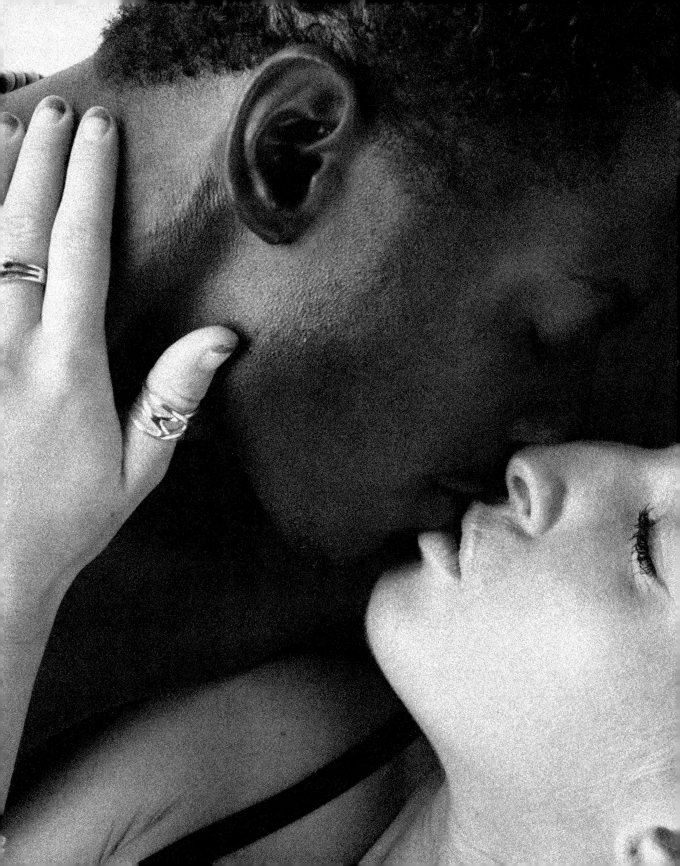

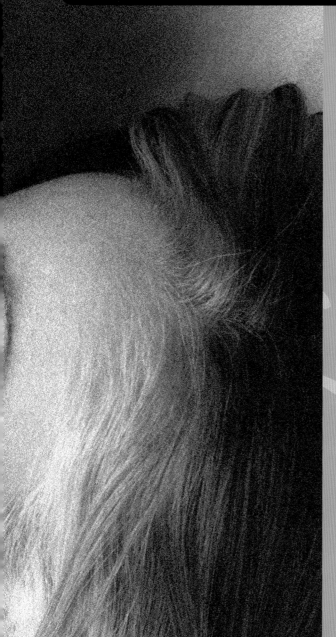

CANCER
JUNE 22 – JULY 22

STAR STATS

Ruling planet MOON
Signature symbol THE CRAB
Metal SILVER
Stone MOONSTONE
Color BLUE

Where to find Cancer Working in banks or the stock market, nosing around DIY stores and antique shops, or running a restaurant.

Hot date Take Cancer to a weepy film (they love a good cry), or just stay at home and snuggle up on the sofa.

Needs and desires Sensitive, sensual, and sexually unpredictable, Cancer needs a mix of physical affection and emotional warmth.

Top turn-on A tongue massage from the top of the spine to down between the buttocks.

Sex positions ♀ The Lotus
♂ Missionary Bliss

Sex toy Shower head or water jets in the swimming pool.

Sex statistic 80 percent of Cancerians are up for sex in the kitchen.

Sensitive, intuitive, and nurturing, the crab is renowned for being moody and unpredictable too. Cancerians have an extraordinary talent for attracting people to them without really trying. But that shy, cautious outer shell hides a highly sexual and sensual lover.

The Moon rules Cancer, and most crabs seem to change their moods and sexual rhythms with the Moon phases. They are never direct about their desires or needs. In fact, they are often sexually and emotionally frustrated because they fear being rejected if they ask for what turns them on. First of all, Cancer needs to feel close, both physically and emotionally. Subtle and sometimes a tad manipulative, crabs approach love and sex in a sideways fashion. They take ages to let you know they're even a little interested but give off all kinds of sensuous signals to sow the right kind of love seeds in your mind. Passively seductive, Cancerians weave their webs slowly and mysteriously, as this makes them feel less vulnerable. They achieve far more through their cool secretiveness, because crabs are looking for complete trust and security before they'll commit themselves to even a first date. The crab often falls for needy people, simply because human weakness and vulnerability is far more interesting to Cancer than strength. Tell Cancer your sad life story and he or she will probably fall in love with you right then and there.

FLIGHTY OR NESTING?

The crab can at times be irritatingly clingy or totally aloof. These changing moods reflect both the crab's need for constant reassurance and fear of rejection. Once Cancerians commit, they usually do so forever and have a great nesting instinct. They hate the thought of emotional dramas, divorce, and separation, and, ironically, that's why they often remain uncommitted or cool off after the first throes of falling in love.

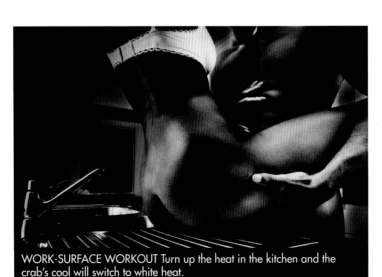
WORK-SURFACE WORKOUT Turn up the heat in the kitchen and the crab's cool will switch to white heat.

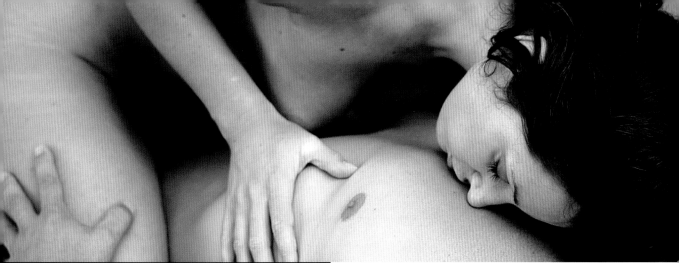

THE CANCER MAN

One of the most complex signs of the zodiac, this sensual but insecure man needs a complicated seduction act too. Crucial to his behavior, the crab has a thing about "mother." Whether it's literally how he feels about his own, or a desire to be mothered by someone, the subject is sure to crop up. He needs to be loved and cherished, but hates to be smothered and has an extraordinary ability to empathize with women and their sensitive nature. However, he doesn't like to admit to his own vulnerable side and can resort to playing a macho role when he can't deal with his moods, feelings, and very needy self. But once he's hooked, he's the ultimate lover. This tender, responsive, and passionate man is one of the true sensualists of the zodiac. However, he is also a very private person, so be warned that he will suddenly retreat into that shell to be alone.

THE CANCER WOMAN

The Cancer woman is enigmatic, funny, warm-hearted, and sexually intuitive. She's the mothering type, but she also wants independence. She seems cool, shy, and unpredictable, but deep down she's passion personified. She wants to

> A sensual **romantic,** Cancer exudes a **sexy** feminine **mystique**

belong to someone, but she hates being possessed. This contradiction of a woman fears opening herself up to rejection, but she is the most loyal and loving of women when she finally commits herself. She needs to be needed and she thrives on closeness.

CANCER IN A NUTSHELL

KEYWORDS Sensitive; sensual; nostalgic; subtle; introspective; moody; emotional; unpredictable; funny

LIKES Caring for others; feeling secure; privacy; being creative; money

DISLIKES Other people messing up the kitchen; possessiveness; taking risks

TRACKING DOWN YOUR CANCER

For all their mystique and emotional undercurrents, crabs are excellent organizers and often hugely ambitious. They may need the odd day of solitude or privacy, but they're easy to track down. More often than not, the crab will be cooking for dinner parties, rummaging at antique fairs, or going shopping.

Cancerians have strong empathy with the past. This gives them a sense of continuity and fills their need for security. Crabs have brilliant memories and an intuitive feeling for what

They are often so fixated on money—theirs and other people's—that they make excellent advisors on stock markets and in investment banking. They have an innate

Small, **intimate** gatherings will help to bring shy Cancerians **out of their shells** and let their innate **social** qualities shine

has worked and what doesn't. They often use their sensitive and caring nature in an industry where their instinct for making sure that people feel good about themselves can lead them to a key managerial or creative role.

MONEY CAN BUY YOU LOVE

Another great place to spot a Cancer is in the world of finance.

nose for collecting fine works of art too. And with their great love of anything from the past, you'll probably find their homes are filled not only with nostalgic old photos and sentimental bits and bobs but also with priceless antiques too. Financial prestige tempts them (along with the security it promises), as do the money industry and expensive, glamorous environments.

MOTHER-LOVE AT WORK

Of course, crabs love their cozy homes more than anything else. But out in the big, wide working world, Cancer naturally wants to "mother" colleagues and treat everyone as part of the family. Secretly ambitious behind that compassionate exterior, they soak up the atmosphere of current trends and the needs of the collective and plan for the future with shrewdness and intuition. Crabs prefer to run things their way rather than be bossed around, and colleagues respect their enterprising spirit.

DINNER PARTIES

If you get invited to a dinner party, then you're sure to meet a Cancer. They prefer small gatherings at home to large events where they can feel quite lost and lonely. But in the kitchen or at a small soirée, they are in their element.

PLACES TO LOOK

BANKS AND FINANCIAL INSTITUTIONS

Money turns them on big time, so check out your local bank or the local supermarket check-out till.

TRUNK SALE

With their love of everything old, Cancerians can always be found nosing around for unusual items at trunk sales, antique shops, or antiquarian bookshops.

RESTAURANTS

Unless they've already become high-class chefs themselves, crabs will thrive on owning or running a restaurant.

THE PARK

Dreamy and caring, the crab will spend hours sitting on a bench feeding the ducks, or playing with a friend or family member's children in the park.

CANCER TOP TEN CAREERS

1 Money-market dealer
2 Banker/Bookkeeper
3 Personnel officer
4 Midwife
5 Historian/Genealogist
6 Archivist
7 Counsellor
8 Hotel manager
9 Women's magazine editor
10 Caterer

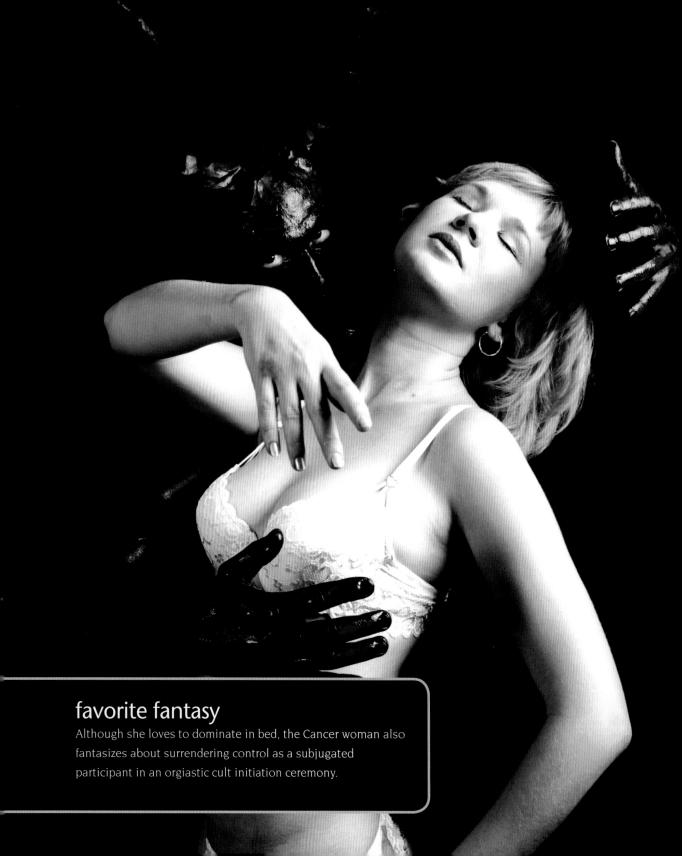

favorite fantasy

Although she loves to dominate in bed, the Cancer woman also
fantasizes about surrendering control as a subjugated
participant in an orgiastic cult initiation ceremony.

WHAT WORKS FOR HER

Cancer's sexual expression is quiet and sultry, yet sexually powerful. Rhythmical, erotic, and feminine, this water sign needs to take her time and slowly dominate. Languid, imaginative arousal is essential in order for her to reach the brink of pulsating passion.

When Cancer gets seriously involved with her lover, her sex drive is on red alert, but there are also times when she'll unconsciously back off, just so she can seduce you all over again. The crab likes to duck and dive in sexual relationships, and not just between the sheets. Subtly manipulative, she actually plays a game that means she's in control of the relationship. Cancer's feelings keep changing, and so does her sexual appetite. She needs a relationship where she has time to retreat to her own private world, but also one where she can be sure

Behind her **shell of reserve,** **intuitive** Cancer is actually one of the most **feminine** and utterly **sensual** women around

of emotional closeness when she's hungry for sex and love.

HOT AND COLD

Basically, she's ultrasensitive to her man's every mood, and her sensual libido can blow hot and cold. But when hot, the lady crab can be the most tender, loving,

passionate, and caring lover. She adores sentimental men who want to know her favorite sex position, kitchen recipe, or the back of her hand in intimate detail. If you've got heart, soul, independent spirit, and might even want a bit of mothering too, then you've met your match.

HOW TO MAKE HER HORNY

Breasts and nipples make Cancer sizzle! This area is the focal point of her zodiac sign's sexual energy flow, which is why good vibrations start here and make for the closest physical and visual contact between you both during foreplay. To turn your watery Cancer lady into a puddle of desire

caress her gently with your fingers in circling movements beneath and around her breasts. Next kiss her between the breasts, making lines of small soft kisses all the way up to the base of her neck and down again. Finally run your tongue slowly around in ever-decreasing circles before stimulating her nipple area with a gentle flicking of your tongue to maximize her arousal

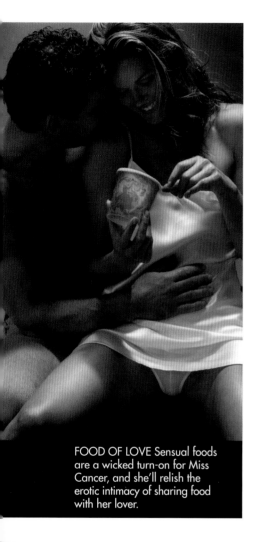

FOOD OF LOVE Sensual foods are a wicked turn-on for Miss Cancer, and she'll relish the erotic intimacy of sharing food with her lover.

SEDUCING THE CRAB

Moon-ruled Cancer is far more of a vamp than she appears on the surface. She hates to be rushed and adores slow, sensual arousal, lingering hands on her belly and breasts, and a refined, exquisite body close to her. Orgasm is like total surrender for her, so trusting in her lover is essential. She is intensely in tune with the vibrations of her arousal and yours, and foreplay must consist of tantalizing sensual stimulation, followed by lots of oral sex.

INSECURE

Undoubtedly, Cancer has many issues around sex and love. She's insecure for one thing, secretly afraid that she will be rejected. And she has a difficult time leaving a man even if she realizes that she may be in the wrong relationship. She demands utter closeness, both physically and emotionally, and if you appear cold or unfeeling, in a hurry, or impatient for orgasm, she'll turn frigid more quickly than water turns to ice in the Arctic. But this is the secret wild-woman of the zodiac, once she's in control of her arousal flow.

EROTICA

Closeness, warmth, and domination are her erotic turn-ons, as well as aphrodisiac foods like oysters, figs, and asparagus. But she's most easily aroused when in the safety of her own bed and hates having sex in places where she doesn't feel comfortable. Share food in her bed, and when you get to know her better, buy her the most erotic lingerie you can find. Once she knows she can truly trust you to stick around, she'll indulge in sex outdoors,

THE LOTUS

Cancer woman has an intuitive sense of giving and receiving orgasmic pleasure, and the Lotus position enhances her responses. To begin, you sit on the floor or bed with legs wide apart. She sits facing you, then clasps her legs around your hips. Now let her slide slowly onto your penis, your hands supporting her buttocks. She loves being in control and setting a languid but powerful sexual rhythm.

THIS FACE-TO-FACE, lovingly entwined position allows for intimate eye contact, deep penetration, and the intense merging of bodies she craves.

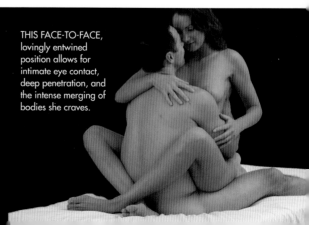

HER TOP TURNOFFS

SUPERFICIALITY
Cancer has no time for idle gossip and anecdotes about your friends. You should be talking about love.

SUBMISSION
She likes to dominate or be your equal. Doggy-style sex, or positions where she doesn't feel physically and emotionally close, will just turn you out of her bed.

EMOTIONAL DISHONESTY
This lady intuitively knows what's going on in your mind and heart just from your body language, so if you can't be honest about your feelings, then forget her.

SAMENESS
Make sure variety is the spice of your crab's sex life. The only thing that's predictable in Cancer's book is the unpredictable.

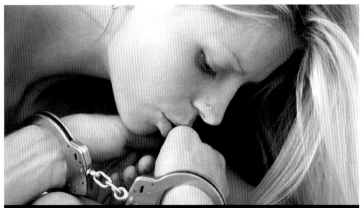

ON TOP OF HER GAME Let your crab dominate in more ways than one: gentle bondage boosts her sex drive. When she's comfortable enough with you to relax her inhibitions, she'll release her wild side.

but opt for sex positions with intense physical closeness and visual contact. She likes to see you orgasm as much as she likes you to see her. For intense, slow arousal, spend time massaging each other with her favorite aromatherapy oil, and tell each other your erotic fantasies.

The Cancer woman secretly loves to imagine she's a dominatrix and will adore gentle bondage scenarios. Let her tie you to the bed with silk scarves, then ask her to suck and tongue your penis to keep you aroused for as long as possible as she masturbates to multiple orgasms. Once she feels totally safe in your hands, she'll adore sitting above your face while you use your tongue and lips to flicker gentle caresses around and into her vulva and vagina.

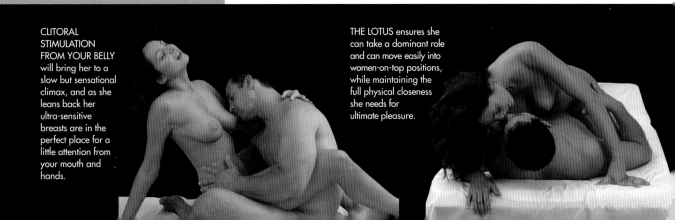

CLITORAL STIMULATION FROM YOUR BELLY will bring her to a slow but sensational climax, and as she leans back her ultra-sensitive breasts are in the perfect place for a little attention from your mouth and hands.

THE LOTUS ensures she can take a dominant role and can move easily into women-on-top positions, while maintaining the full physical closeness she needs for ultimate pleasure.

WHAT WORKS FOR HIM

Careful now: he may appear cool, undemanding, and serene, but beneath that subtle approach this man is smolderingly sensual with a sizzling sex drive. And the good news is that he really wants to make sure he can adapt to your rhythms and sexual needs too.

The sensual Cancer man is an old-style romantic when it comes to wooing women

Cancer doesn't like loudmouthed, direct women. He's turned on by feminine mystique, self-reliance, and emotional honesty. A true sensualist, he adores all the trappings of languid romance: candles, home-cooked meals, and cuddling up on sofas together. Hand-holding in the park, kissing in the dark at the cinema, or in the back of the taxi. He'll love the lingering smell of your perfume on his shirtsleeve and gaze at your phone number while he's working in the office. In fact, he sounds like a bit of an easy catch. But to seduce him you need to feed him romantic carrots, such as "I've never felt like this before", one day, then the next, "I'm off to see my friends," which proves you're committed but will give him time and space to be alone.

EMOTIONAL NEEDS

The Cancer man finds it difficult to accept he has feelings and sometimes will act the macho man to get what he wants. He can be manipulative and play all kinds of emotional games just to get you in his bed, then drop you just as quickly to avoid entangling those "feelings." But deep down he can be needy, and once he's secure in your arms, he can also act like clingwrap.

HOW TO MAKE HIM HORNY

Slow, sensual movements and five-star face-to-face closeness brings the crab out of his shell and gets him scuttling toward the bedroom. However, you do need to take your time and treat making love like a work of art. His torso, chest, and nipples are his primary astro-erogenous zone, so sit astride him and kiss his belly and chest all over. Trace your fingers around his sensitive nipples and then finger them gently until they are erect. Run your tongue around the outside of his nipples and suck on them, then kiss him deeply, tongue literally in cheek, and he'll be begging for more. Take things to the next level by rubbing your breasts and nipples sensuously across his chest and belly: the closer the contact is between your torso and belly and his, the more aroused he'll get.

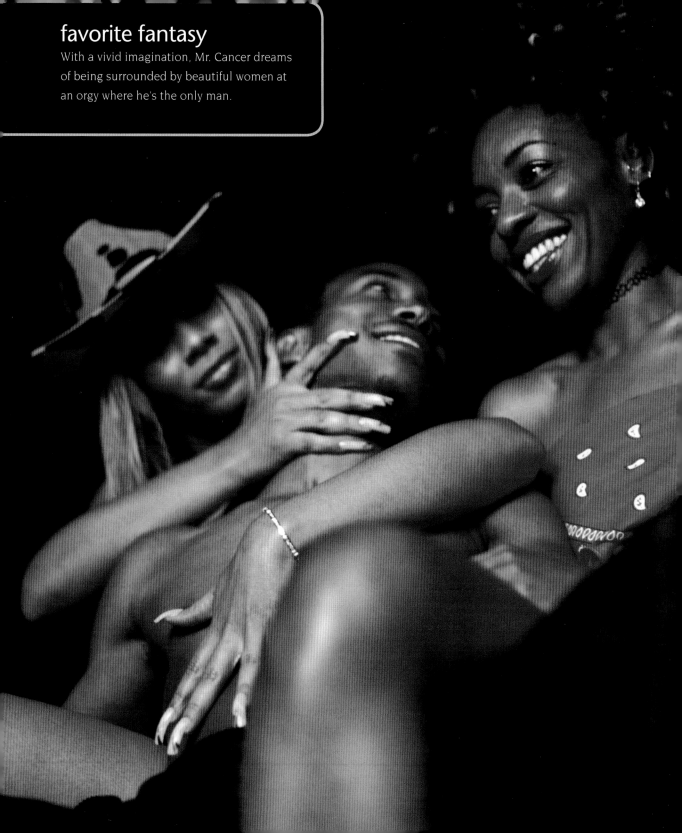

favorite fantasy

With a vivid imagination, Mr. Cancer dreams of being surrounded by beautiful women at an orgy where he's the only man.

CARING AND LOYAL

He cares, he really does, but remember that his libido swings from high to low. If you catch him when he's feeling horny, he's the most tender, rampant, and sensual of lovers. He's not into direct, aggressive, or crazy sex. He may have a hot body and sophistication to match, but he does have feelings too. Orgasm for him is about emotional closeness as well as just having sex for the fun of it. And the Cancer man often has a problem ejaculating because he fears his vulnerability will be on show. On the other hand, he really cares about your sexual needs and will sacrifice his own to make sure you're in orgasmic bliss.

ROLE-PLAYER

He's a real sensualist but needs a high fantasy or role-playing turn-on to match. Pretend you're in a historical drama. Let him be whoever he chooses—anyone from Casanova to a pharaoh or a business tycoon. His best buzz is when he's being dominated. And oral sex comes high on his priorities. In fact, it's often more of a turn-on for him than sexual intercourse, and puts off the feeling of guilt that is generated from a deep-seated complex about "incest with mother."

To get him relaxed and free from inhibitions, suggest you take the lead and gently tie his hands to a chair with silk scarves while he's naked. Run your fingers all over his body until he's tingling, then do the same with your lips. Then your nipples. Serve dinner naked to whet his appetite. Be dressed as a vamp, then make love to him with only your stilettos on.

Water is a sensational turn-on that will make him do anything

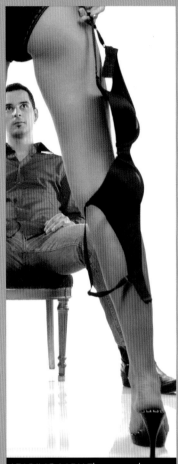

LEADING LADY The sensual and imaginative Cancer man will quickly rise to any vampish bait.

MISSIONARY BLISS

In all its variations, the man-on-top Missionary provides exactly the physical closeness and comfort of seeing you as "his" in all your glory that the Cancer man craves. Although he likes to be dominated eventually, this old favorite gives him an immediate feeling of security. From the basic position, it is easy to introduce variants and switch roles.

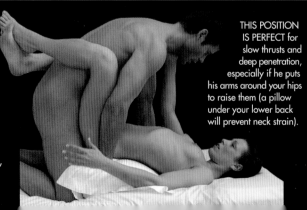

THIS POSITION IS PERFECT for slow thrusts and deep penetration, especially if he puts his arms around your hips to raise them (a pillow under your lower back will prevent neck strain).

you ask. Indulge in lengthy foreplay and you'll realize he's the master of oral sex. Take a bath together and massage his penis in the bubbles as he lies between your legs. Swap places and masturbate yourself, then sit astride him and have sex

mother figure, or someone to "mother," rather than a lover and partner who is an equal. Security conscious, once involved, the crab finds it very hard to let go. The same goes for sex. Once he establishes a tried and trusted method or sex

> His **sensuality** might surprise you once you've **got over** the barrier of his **inhibitions**

in the tub. Ask him to be your sex slave, as submission keeps him craving more. With your dress on, ask him to give you oral sex while you're standing up and he's totally naked.

MOTHER LOVE

Cancer men are frequently unconsciously looking for a

position, he often sticks to that rather than try new or "risky" things. To free him from this "safe" circle of habitual response, you'll have to work very slowly on showing him new techniques. Introduce racy doggy-style positions and anal sex only if you've known him a long time.

HIS TOP TURNOFFS

COOLNESS
Get warm. If you're the kind of woman who spends more time in the bathroom than in his bed, he'll just pull the plug on the relationship.

FRIVOLITY
The crab can't bear gossipy, two-faced women. Be emotional, ask for support, tell him your problems and he's truly caring; turn to your social life and he couldn't care a bit.

MATERIAL INSECURITY
He hates feeling insecure about money. If you haven't got any, don't mention it.

WOMEN'S LIBBERS
He does like independence and equality of the sexes, but not freedom fighters.

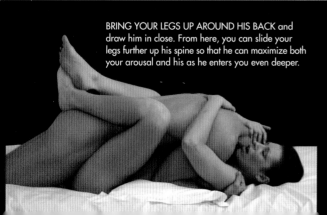

BRING YOUR LEGS UP AROUND HIS BACK and draw him in close. From here, you can slide your legs further up his spine so that he can maximize both your arousal and his as he enters you even deeper.

NOW ROLL OVER TO SIT ASTRIDE HIM in Missionary style. You can increase the sense of closeness by moving your legs down either side of him for a full-body embrace.

IS THIS THE ONE?

Crabs want emotional peace and long-term commitment. However, they often fall into the wrong relationship and then fear trying to leave. But if you are kind, compassionate, and loyal, they make tender and trusting partners.

ARIES AND CANCER

The ram's passion is wild and totally indiscreet; the crab's is clandestine and secret. Words like commitment and security send the ram running. Great for a passionate affair, but the crab's feelings aren't what interests Aries, only Aries does.

TAURUS AND CANCER

An easy-going lifestyle, because neither wants to score points over the other. Cancer empathizes with the bull's security-conscious nature, and loves those cozy nights in. A sense of stability guaranteed as long as both really want to be there.

GEMINI AND CANCER

Gemini lives in the mind, the crab in feelings. But you're both restless souls, and your unpredictable relationship tactics amuse each other. But Gemini's after freedom, not dependence, so not easy if Cancer wants commitment.

CANCER AND CANCER

You both fear rejection more than anything else, so opening up to each other could take a long time. In fact, your romantic tango could carry on longer than most other relationships. You're both quite needy, and this can lead to manipulative games.

LEO AND CANCER

Strangely, often a good match. Flamboyant and impulsive, Leos are demanding but Cancers love to mother them. Sexually addictive, Leo adores the crab's protectiveness and Cancer loves to be loved. This could be an utterly devoted duo.

VIRGO AND CANCER

Meticulous beyond belief, Virgo believes that what you see is what you get, while Cancer doesn't and believes in mystery. Both feel deeply but rarely open up. Fascinating sexual rapport, but can lead to misunderstanding in practical affairs.

Cancer will initially respond eagerly to Libra's idealistic vision of love, and Libra will adore the crab's sensitive, sensual nature. But eventually Libra's lofty, abstract approach to life may not sit well in Cancer's emotional world. More lows than highs.

LIBRA AND CANCER

Usually an erotic and deeply emotional relationship, both aware of the other's sexual energy flow. However, Scorpio wants to control all aspects of the relationship, and Cancer needs unpredictability and privacy. Potentially destructive.

SCORPIO AND CANCER

Short-lived but memorable. Cancer's home-loving, but the archer isn't exactly fond of leaning over a hot stove. Magnetic sexually, but Sagittarius wants freedom and a nomadic lifestyle while Cancer needs commitment and a nest.

SAGITTARIUS AND CANCER

Serious sexy rapport and often highly successful. Capricorns will take a while to break through Cancer's defensive boundaries, but once you've proved that you're there for life, you probably will be. Better if both are ambitious about work.

CAPRICORN AND CANCER

Could be a stimulating sexual relationship, but Cancer will get jealous of all Aquarius's exes turning up as friends. Fascinated by each other's different sexuality, but Cancer gets needy, and Aquarius won't play mother for long.

AQUARIUS AND CANCER

Have an intuitive understanding of each other's feelings and sexual needs. Pisces knows how to please, and Cancer loves taking pleasure. A very private relationship, but Cancer will have to make the decisions if they're to get out of the house.

PISCES AND CANCER

AND THE WINNER IS...

The other two water signs, Scorpio and Pisces, are highly favorable combinations with Cancer. They both respond through their feeling world, and this makes Cancer feel an immediate sense of belonging. However, crabs really need someone who can support them through thick and thin, indulge them in their love of the past, and languid, sensual sexuality, and enjoy a tranquil home life. So if there's a real winner, then Taurus is streets ahead of the rest of the signs. Both are security conscious, loving comfort and the good things of life, and can build a secure, loving relationship together.

LONG-TERM LOVE WITH CANCER

Moody and acutely sensitive, Cancer is one of the more complex signs of the zodiac. But crabs offer utter devotion, sensual savvy, and an instinctive understanding of your deepest feelings. If you're looking for an exquisite lover who is also a secure homemaker and offers long-term commitment, then Cancer is the one for you.

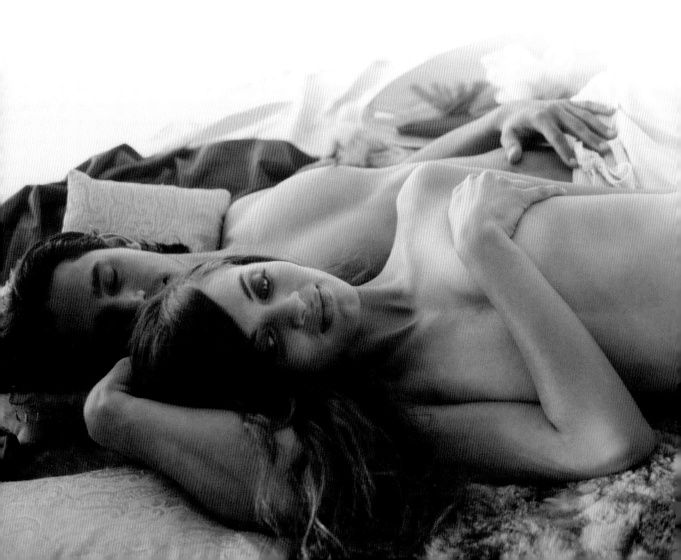

Cancer thrives on being needed, both sexually and emotionally. However, although crabs can be inconsistent and terribly needy themselves, if you go with the flow of their feelings and don't take things too personally when they retreat into their shells, then they will be loyal and imaginative partners both in bed and out of it. But don't take Cancerians for granted: they may be sensitive and clingy, but they can see right through emotional dishonesty.

commitment, and together you can create a stylish and secure home to satisfy the crab's nesting instinct into the bargain.

HABIT FORMING

Cancerians are creatures of habit. They feel safe when they know what to expect from you and that you'll always be there for them. So although the crab might do everything in a totally illogical and roundabout way, if you can be a rock of strength

PEELING OFF THE CLINGWRAP

The crab does get very clingy and can be quite hard to shake off, so if you want to get a Cancerian to ditch you, then you'll have to play a very subtle game. The trick is to criticize them openly in public, and simultaneously turn off the affection in private. Pretty soon they'll get this feeling that you can't satisfy their neediness anymore and will scuttle away to look for someone else to, well, cling to.

> Cancer is oh-so **responsive** to **tender caresses**, gentle lovemaking, and sharing **mutual dreams** for the future

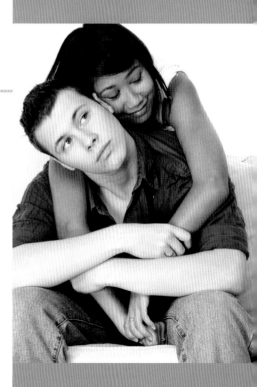

COMMITMENT

Be affectionate and dedicated to the crab's creative talents, but have a career of your own. Be prepared to change plans at the drop of a hat and Cancer will put all his or her trust in you. To keep your crab happy, you must also be sympathetic to his or her fears and woes, be a good listener and be as cautious about money as he or she is. Then he or she'll reward you with deep and long-lasting

and be the consistent force in his or her life, together you'll create a genuine long-lasting and deeply bonding partnership. Encourage Cancerians to come out of their shells when they feel down, and they'll do everything in their power to help you to the top of your profession or just sincerely empathize with your troubles. Never underestimate the crab's desire to make this relationship a habit of a lifetime.

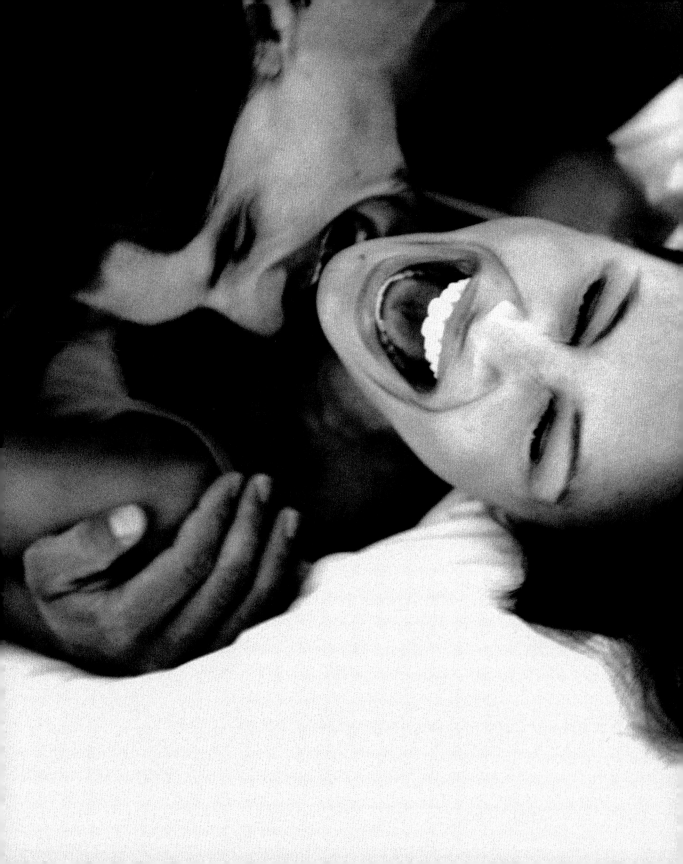

LEO

JULY 23 – AUGUST 23

STAR STATS

Ruling planet SUN
Signature symbol THE LION
Metal GOLD
Stone DIAMOND
Color ORANGE

Where to find Leo On a stage or film set, in glamorous restaurants and shops, or luxurious hotels and resorts.

Hot date The most exclusive nightclub where celebs hang out.

Needs and desires Fiery and extravagant, flamboyant Leo needs a loyal and down-to-earth lover who's also open-minded about Leo's exhibitionist streak.

Top turn-on Visual arousal. Have sex in the daytime, or watch each other orgasm by candlelight.

Sex positions ♀ The Top
♂ King of the Jungle

Sex toy Fluffy rug.

Sex statistic 88 percent of Leos have sex on their mind 88 percent of the day.

WHAT TO EXPECT WITH LEO

Fiery Leo, the roaring lion of the zodiac demands to be treated like royalty. They adore being center stage, have high expectations of relationships, yet always give their all to the ones they love. Proud and glamorous, they are the sexually charged monarchs of the zodiac.

The Sun rules Leo and is the source of all life on earth. And, likewise, Leos insist on being number one, fanning the flames of love and romance for as long as possible. Vain, flamboyant, and theatrical, they love to put on a show or act a part. They're never short of admirers, and they exude unlimited passion and a fiery sexuality.

SPECIAL

Sounds like the perfect partner? Well, up to a point. But the point is that Leos are suckers for fame, power, money, status, and "who you know." And that's fine if you happen to have rich friends or family, are of A-list social status, or have a fabulous career. Not so good if you're a shelf-filler. Leo needs a classy partner who shimmers at social events and is a bit of a snob. In fact, Leos are secretly insecure about their specialness. So the more important they think you are, the more attracted they'll be to you, and with you propping up their image, the more they'll feel happy about themselves.

HIGH EXPECTATIONS

Leos can be the most loyal partners and lovers, if you can live up to their heady ideal of eternal romance and their demanding grandiosity. Not easy. Leos' greatest qualities of magnanimous attention and generosity often get distorted if their lovers start to take more of an interest in themselves. And Leos always think they're right, and they just won't take no for an answer. However, if you can flatter, flirt, and keep the romance and sex going in Leo's favor 24/7, then the lion will proudly be your mate for life.

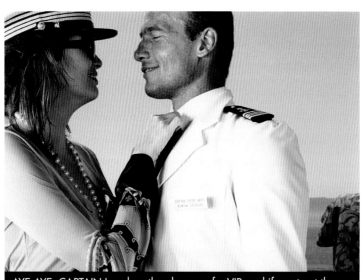

AYE AYE, CAPTAIN Leos love the glamour of a VIP, and if you treat them like one too, they'll be putty in your hands.

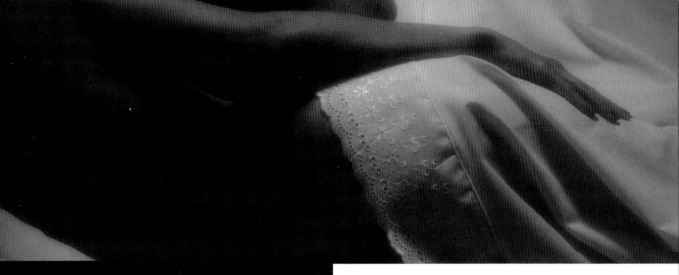

THE LEO MAN

He wants to feel like a king and be adored for his cheeky sexiness. He can't imagine ever being turned down, and matched with his charisma it's the kind of assumption that will make you say

> He can appear **cocky** but if you **stroke** that **ego** he'll **purr**

"yes, more, more!" Ultimately, the Leo man can be a tad macho. If you draw the crowds first, that's fine, but he'll want to take over the limelight. This man seeks a perfect princess to play an outstanding supporting role to the main actor—himself.

THE LEO WOMAN

The lioness of the zodiac has to be the center of the universe in her partner's eyes. The more adored she is, the more aroused she'll get. But she also needs someone who has no inhibitions about being dominated, enjoys the odd drama and pillow fight in the bedroom, and is equally passionate about exhibitionist sex. What she wants more than anything else is a glamorous relationship with a man who knows how to give her a good time. Everything counts and has to be of the highest quality: romance, luxury items, delicious meals, social whirls. Luxury and fame and all the glitz make her feel loved and *numero uno*. Showbiz is what the Leo woman is about, but beneath the flashy exterior, the lioness has a soft heart. She needs to learn that no one in the world is perfect, not even herself.

LEO IN A NUTSHELL

KEYWORDS Fiery; dramatic; vain; immature; romantic; stylish; flamboyant; demanding; self-centered; excessive

LIKES Money and a fan club; role-playing; exaggerated flattery; glamour

DISLIKES Routines; responsibilities; being ignored; rivals; reality

TRACKING DOWN YOUR LEO

Leos want to be the stars of the show, so you won't have much trouble tracking them down: they're the ones holding court in the middle of a social event, or up on the stage in the limelight. They love being spotted in all the trendiest places, so head for the stylish nightspot that everyone wants to be seen in.

Leos believe they deserve the best, because they believe they are the best. (This is sometimes a compensation for a big chip on their shoulders.) So obviously where you'll find them is getting hotel bar where someone famous once visited, sardined at the front of a rock concert, or running the local opera group, Leo must truly keep up with the glamour and glitz of life.

You'll find Leo **center stage,** not blending in, so head for the **bright lights** and look for the person **holding court**

as near to the rich and famous as possible, if they're not a local celebrity themselves. They love shopping for luxury goods, and spend hours choosing new outfits, window-shopping when they're feeling a little skint, bargain-hunting on the Internet, and showing off their latest new "must-have" item in the swish coffee shop in their lunch hour. Whether sipping a cocktail in a

STAGE AND SCREEN

Flamboyant and focused, Leos need to be in a position where they can control and reign like royalty. If they're not the star of the show, they'll unleash a fiery self-confidence to get them to the top and beat their competitors. Leos thrive on future possibilities rather than worrying about past mistakes. They often become highly successful business entrepreneurs because they love to take charge. As long as they're on some kind of throne or stage surrounded by admirers, they soar, delegate, and always look like they've made a million bucks, even if they haven't. The arts, film, theater, and the teaching professions provide Leos with a medium for expressing their flair for drama or acting out a role.

THE DANCE FLOOR

They may not make ballroom-dancing champions, but they try hard to live up to that kind of image. You'll find them beneath the dazzling lights of any dance floor. As disco-fever king or queen, salsa expert or tango maestro, Leos love to show off their charisma. They also enjoy posing in gyms, sports arenas, and on beaches, but they won't be the ones working up a sweat. You'll spot Leos strutting their stuff, not suffering for their art!

PLACES TO LOOK

NIGHTCLUB
Surrounded by admirers at the bar, Leos adore the glitz and glamour of the small hours.

THEATER
If they're not on stage, they'll be working as director, agent, or producer. Film and stage schools have a high percentage of talented Leos wanting fame.

ART GALLERY
Either they've got an exhibition on or they swan around galleries admiring stylish modern or classic art. Leos have incredible creative talent if they acknowledge it.

BOARDROOM
Leos who don't unleash their creative talents on the world usually end up running the show. They often chair the board, indulging in office politics.

LEO TOP TEN CAREERS

1 Actor/Singer
2 Entertainer
3 Exhibitions organizer
4 Film director/Working in films
5 Teacher
6 Theatrical agent
7 Stockbroker
8 Educational advisor
9 Obstetrician
10 Creative director

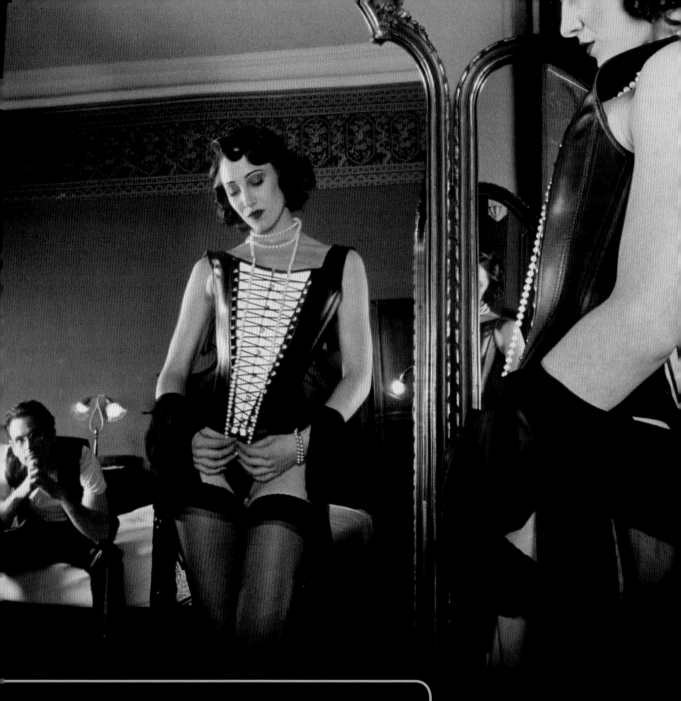

favorite fantasy

Exhibitionist Miss Leo loves performing to an audience and
fantasizes about masturbating herself in front of mirrors with
a voyeur discovering her in the moment of orgasm.

WHAT WORKS FOR HER

Intensely individual, the lioness of the zodiac knows she's desirable and must have a dramatic love life to match her theatrical image. Her sexual style is flamboyant and dominating and she seduces with all the wiles of a wildcat. Treat her like royalty, and she'll be yours forever.

Miss Leo seeks men who will go wild with admiration for her. She craves privileged treatment and the best possible arm to hang on in public. And if her partner can keep up with that permanent twinkle in her eye, she'll be up for raunchy sex in public places and behind closed doors. To get her attention, be a little ego-centric yourself, and show you have a large reserve of money, or at least know how to save it.

> Just like a **lioness**, she's fiercely **territorial**—once she's set her eyes on you, you're **hers**, and it's **all or nothing**

ALL OR NOTHING

Demanding though she can be, Leo is hugely creative with her sexual and romantic passion and loves to make dramatic gestures like driving through a storm just to be in your arms. She wants to prove she's the best lover, and often goes out of her way to perform daring or crazy sexual antics. However, the lioness is also very shrewd about getting what she wants, and does so with theatrical confidence. Leos have been known to push aside rivals like a drama queen, and get to the front of the line for some handsome hunk who's notorious for penis size and sexual flair.

HOW TO MAKE HER HORNY

Leo's sexual energy flow has its epicenter down the length of her spine. Target this area even when you are first kissing face-to-face by including light, teasing strokes up and down this astro-erogenous zone, first through her clothing, then over bare skin. Enhance her pleasure further by running your fingers down her back and gently massaging each bone of her spine in turn (be very careful when working directly on the spine). She'll have fantastic surges of adrenaline-packed pleasure if you slowly lick along her spine starting at the nape of her neck, right down to the cleft between her buttocks. By now, your sultry lioness should be purring like a kitten. As a variant, in the middle of a steamy sex session, try sitting astride her back and rubbing your penis along her spine for tingling sex-sational results.

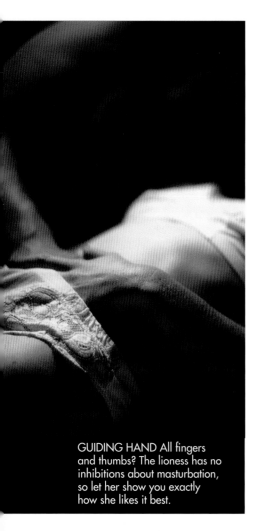

GUIDING HAND All fingers and thumbs? The lioness has no inhibitions about masturbation, so let her show you exactly how she likes it best.

DRAMA QUEEN

The Leo woman's sexual expression is dazzling and fiery. Not afraid of asking for exactly what she wants, Leo is direct and honest about her sexual needs and demands total adoration. (You must have eyes for her body only.) She loves all the glamorous accoutrements of sex, as well as provocative foreplay and teasing touches. She enjoys clitoral stimulation while fully clothed or the rub of leather against her inner thigh.

Outrageous and self-important, Leo flaunts and indulges in her pleasure. Sex is a complete theatrical performance where she takes center stage. The Top is the perfect position to start the ball rolling. This technique also gives her maximum visual stimulation, aligning with her need for exhibitionist arousal and stylish climax. You can then follow through with other more physically demanding positions like the Eagle (see pages 22–23), which will unleash her need to dominate and take total control, or the Tiger (see pages 166–67) to intensify orgasm.

Treating her as though she's famous is enough to give her a real sexual high. But you've got to be classy, act as though you're a celebrity and make her feel like the most special woman on earth in the first five minutes of sex.

FIERY EGOTIST

The lioness's erotic triggers are all about her being the center of attention. So taking control is a very potent turn-on for her. Sophisticated bondage (let her bind you to the bed with lace or silk scarves) and exhibitionist sex are also great adrenaline arousers, especially if you can get away with doing something in a

THE TOP

This theatrical position is a showstopper for your exhibitionist lioness. In theory, she revolves a full 360° on top of you, but completing the turn without the penis slipping out will take a lot of practice—lucky for both of you! The varying views and sensations are very exciting and satisfy her need for visual arousal, and she will adore the sexy sense of control that the position gives her.

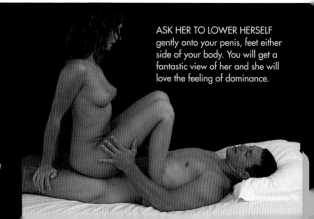

ASK HER TO LOWER HERSELF gently onto your penis, feet either side of your body. You will get a fantastic view of her and she will love the feeling of dominance.

HER TOP TURNOFFS

SOFTIES

If you're just pretending to be a macho man when in reality you can't keep up with her rampant sex drive, it'll be a swift good-bye from the lioness.

CHEAP PRESENTS

Leo believes she deserves luxury, not bargains or tat. So make sure that you always buy her the most expensive perfumes, accessories, or sexy lingerie. If you can't provide her with the best, she'll find someone who can.

BEING TOLD WHAT TO DO

Leo is a bit like a naughty child: she likes to play up, tease, and provoke. But if you try to stop her, she'll simply pick up her toys and go play somewhere else. This is one female who'll never admit that you know best.

public place as well. The dare factor gives her a real libido boost, and she's likely to suggest anything from foreplay in the back of the taxi to penetrative sex in a classy nightclub restroom. The more outrageous the location, the more orgasms she'll have.

Suggest she rips off your clothes while standing face-to-face. Then let her play with her nipples and breasts in front of you without you touching. Watch yourselves in a mirror as you masturbate simultaneously, or as she kneels and gives you a blowjob, then swap roles. Indulge in erotic or pornographic movies together, and then perform the same moves and techniques.

VISUAL TREAT

Leo loves to see herself in action, or to imagine she's showing off her sexual know-how in front of an audience,

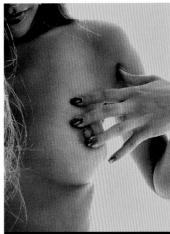

NIPPLE PLAY Miss Leo adores showing off her breasts and teasing you with her erect nipples, so enjoy the private viewing!

so make love in front of mirrors. Oral sex especially gives her a sense of power and control over the sexual performance, but she needs to learn that her partner also has a right to express his individual sexual needs, and that for all her fiery egotism, she's acutely feminine too.

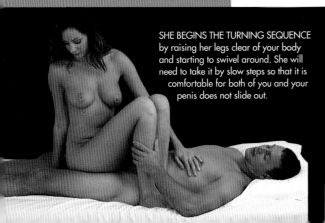

SHE BEGINS THE TURNING SEQUENCE by raising her legs clear of your body and starting to swivel around. She will need to take it by slow steps so that it is comfortable for both of you and your penis does not slide out.

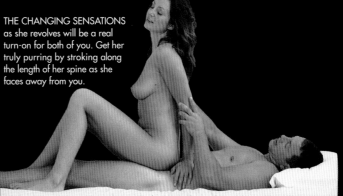

THE CHANGING SENSATIONS as she revolves will be a real turn-on for both of you. Get her truly purring by stroking along the length of her spine as she faces away from you.

WHAT WORKS FOR HIM

Sex for Mr. Leo is "now or never." He's got the passion, the uninhibited performance, and the spontaneous sex drive usually on red alert all day and night. He's aroused quickly, and there's nothing that will stop him having you when he's in the mood. Quite frankly, he wants sex whenever he can get it.

> Leo's **optimism** and lust for life are truly **infectious**, and once he's decided you're **worth it**, he'll include you in **all the fun**

Now if the lion sounds like a walking sex bomb, that's because he is. But he does have feelings despite all that self-importance. The benevolent dictator of the zodiac really has a heart, but he's also vain and showy, cocky and demanding. And he's so arrogant that he assumes he won't be turned down. He zooms in with persuasion, seduction, and deliberate drama to see if he can turn you into a quivering wreck. If he can, then you're not worthy of his regal passion, but if he can't, then maybe—just maybe—you might be his kind of princess. Once he starts whirling you around the dance floor or letting you hang on his arm at every social event, it's a statement that you're part of his kingdom.

JOY STICK

With a wildly insatiable libido, his performance is extreme, larger than life, or just large. Don't ever assume you're the star of the show, sexual or otherwise. This is Mr. Ego with a big penis, and he'll rarely share his limelight with a woman who is more dramatic than he is.

HOW TO MAKE HIM HORNY

Mr. Leo's astro-erogenous zone is located between his shoulder blades and down his spine. Start off by running your fingernails across his back in zig-zag fashion so he doesn't know which direction you're going in next—the uncertainty will make the sensations all the more erotic—then gently kiss him between his shoulder blades. To raise the temperature still further, run your tongue down his spine and then back up again, being careful not to reach as far as the cleft of his buttocks. Follow this up with dabbing and flickering movements of your tongue across his back and then down the sides of his torso. Now go for the direct approach: push your hand beneath him and feel his penis hard and ready for action. After that, it's up to him. Remember, this lion is the king of the jungle!

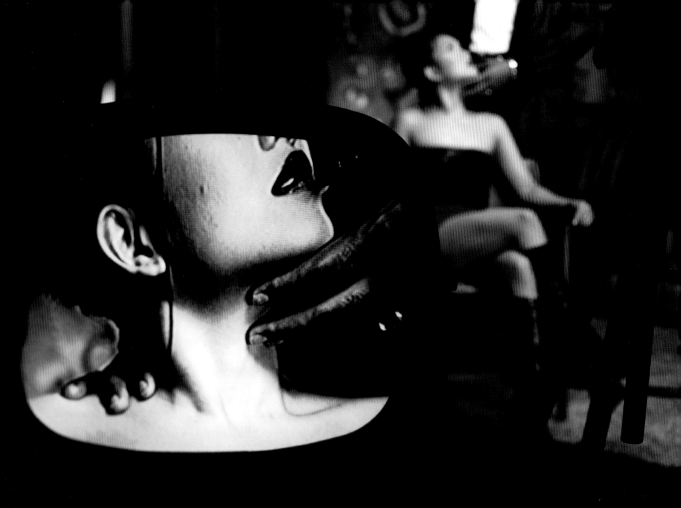

favorite fantasy

Mr. Leo likes to take charge in the bedroom, and loves the idea of having a courtesan, geisha, or virgin slaving to his every whim in front of a camera.

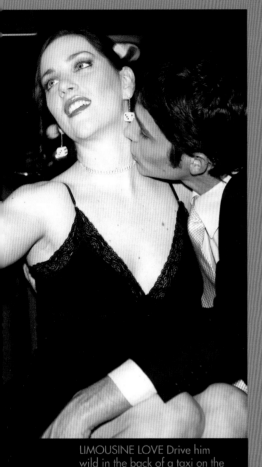

LIMOUSINE LOVE Drive him wild in the back of a taxi on the way home and his sex drive will be on red alert all night.

LION KING

He's convinced he knows the only way to turn you on or that his favorite techniques are more important than yours. Two stars are one too many. He's the ultimate in lust drive, so never complain, criticize, or make fun of him, or you'll be forgotten on the spot. But if you're up for pure, undiluted lust and a potent performance, then this man is unmatchable. And lust for Leo equates with romance.

FRAGILE EGO

Known for being one of the most sexually "active" signs of the zodiac, Mr. Leo really wants a partner who gives him that "wow" factor. He expects the best and has high standards to keep up, for both his sexual performance and yours. If you're not ready to play his games, or resort to your fantasy world, Leo can roar with criticism or become distant, with his pride wounded and his ego chipped. He often projects mythical qualities onto his lover, expecting her to be as special and superhuman as he is, and can react badly when she doesn't live up to this image. If you don't regularly boost his ego and sexual esteem, he'll quickly find a new lioness to hang on his arm.

PERFECT PERFORMANCE

In spite of his rapid arousal, his pace is slow. There's a steady build-up of sexual energy that means you must align your sexual rhythm with his. He has to be in control, and the stage must be set with luxurious accoutrements like fine wine, sex toys, satin sheets, foaming baths, or gold candles. Leo doesn't have a big thing about kissing, and often prefers just to get on with oral sex when he

KING OF THE JUNGLE

Regal Mr. Leo prefers a position where he's dominant, to begin with anyway (when he feels that he can trust you, he might let you take a turn as well). He loves to utterly throw himself into hard, pumping intercourse, with a partner who appreciates him. Face-to-face sex is a great way for Leo to "see" what's going on. After all, it's not so much the touchy-feely stuff that turns him on but visual stimulation.

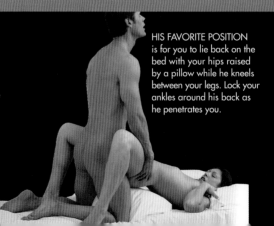

HIS FAVORITE POSITION is for you to lie back on the bed with your hips raised by a pillow while he kneels between your legs. Lock your ankles around his back as he penetrates you.

chooses. He believes that he can satisfy any woman, and takes great pride in his sexual prowess.

EXHIBITIONIST

Glamour and power are big turn-ons. Dress in vampish clothes and then make him up with your favorite cosmetics. Use eyeliner, lipsticks, or fake tattoos and make a work of art of his face, his belly, and his inner thighs. He's an exhibitionist, so take photos of him nude, in arty sexy positions and lighting. By the time you've finished he'll want you as his sex slave. Mutual masturbation is an instant arouser, particularly if it's in a public place, like the back of a taxi, the cinema, or even in a bar or restaurant, discreetly beneath the table.

Have sex in front of mirrors or cameras. Seeing himself in action is his prime arousal and means he'll give as good as he gets.

> He's more **concerned** with his climax than **yours**, so gently **remind him** of your needs

Position a video camera in your bedroom and tell him he's a film director who's been seduced by the leading lady. Use your feet and breasts to stimulate his penis, rub oils into his body, and then give him the best blow job ever. Ask him to masturbate you in front of a mirror and then watch as you orgasm together.

HIS TOP TURNOFFS

NEGLECT
He must be the center of attention. Tell him he's the best lover since sliced bread or you won't be sharing his toast in the morning.

SLOPPY DRESSERS
He wants you to be the perfect princess. If you yawn about life, drink tea instead of champagne, or wear old jeans when you could dress to kill, think again.

UNCONVENTIONAL SEX
Exhibitionist he may be, but Mr. Leo likes tried and trusted methods of orgasm. If you're up for S&M, threesomes, or anal sex, your lion will find another pride.

COMPETITION
He's totally turned off by women who want to compete with him in bed or out of it.

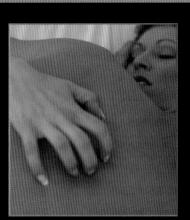

HIS ASTRO-EROGENOUS ZONE is centered around his shoulder blades, so he'll love it if you show your claws a little and gently rake this area as he leans over you.

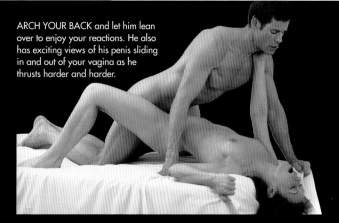

ARCH YOUR BACK and let him lean over to enjoy your reactions. He also has exciting views of his penis sliding in and out of your vagina as he thrusts harder and harder.

IS THIS THE ONE?

Leos have such high expectations of love and sex that it's difficult for anyone to live up to the divine image of their long-term mate. However, there are a few signs of the zodiac who can take pride of place in Leo's very warm heart.

ARIES AND LEO

You're both vain and Aries is impulsive. A competitive edge both sexually and materially, which can be exhausting, and your fiery enthusiasm can burn itself out. Each quickly tires of the other's company: great for a fling, but not easy long-term.

TAURUS AND LEO

The bull is a sensual artist but doesn't aspire to flamboyance. Leo makes a drama out of life; Taurus prefers working quietly behind the scenes. Fascinated by each other's differences to begin with, Taurus won't satisfy Leo's need for attention.

GEMINI AND LEO

The lion lives with the heart, Gemini with the head. You entertain each other, but the twins' inconsistent and flirtatious nature will drive Leo mad. Very unstable, and Gemini won't match up to Leo's demanding standards for long.

CANCER AND LEO

Unexpectedly, often an excellent rapport. Cancer is inspired by Leo's fiery outgoing nature and genuinely wants Leo to feel ultra special. A truly passionate love affair, but Cancer needs to stay at home while Leo wants to socialize.

LEO AND LEO

Obviously have a lot in common, but this quickly becomes a battle of stubborn wills. A great sexual power game is being played and it can produce spectacular fireworks. You're both so proud; if you've made a mistake you'll never admit it.

VIRGO AND LEO

Virgo easily relates to the lion's high standards of beauty, sexuality, and polished performance. But Leos will get resentful when Virgos think they always know all the answers. A creative relationship if you can respect each other's different approaches.

Both love to get out and about, look good, and enjoy a glittering social life, but Libra's indecisiveness will eventually irritate Leo. Wonderful for sexy fun and mutual adoration, but hard to pin each other down to long-term plans.

LIBRA AND LEO

A passionate, often off-and-on relationship based on sexual and emotional power games. Leo is showy, teasing, and glamorous, Scorpio smoldering and difficult to satisfy. If Leo's social life doesn't make Scorpio jealous, it could last.

SCORPIO AND LEO

Dynamic and romantic, sexually you get on like a house on fire. But poor long-term prospects. Sagittarius prefers freedom and isn't terribly loyal in the sex department. Leo is too controlling and the archer's an incurable roamer.

SAGITTARIUS AND LEO

An exciting rapport, dramatic and erotic, often making for a steamy relationship. Leo falls for the goat's classy libido, and Capricorn loves the lion's outrageous sexuality. A workable relationship, if you can sort out who's the boss.

CAPRICORN AND LEO

Difficult but tantalizing between opposite signs of the zodiac. Leo believes in exclusive love, Aquarius in nonexclusive relationships. The lion's proud and self-indulgent; Aquarius is detached and worries about the world. Hard to sustain.

AQUARIUS AND LEO

Great for escapism, romance, and intrigue, but not easy long-term. Fantasy and drama interweave sexually, but fixed fire and mutable water have very different outlooks on life. The fish might fall for the romance rather than the real Leo.

PISCES AND LEO

AND THE WINNER IS...

Although the other two fire signs, Aries and Sagittarius, can empathize with Leo's flamboyant world, they'll clash when it comes to that thing about exclusivity. Leo will enjoy romancing and socializing with Libra and playing power games with Scorpio. If one sign has to win out in the end, then Capricorn is probably the only sign who aspires to the same stylish and luxurious lifestyle that Leos demand, and who can give them a real run for their money.

LONG-TERM LOVE WITH LEO

The lion is not only a proud fire sign but a fixed one too, and that means they are searching for a permanent partnership. Generous and flamboyant, once they realize you won't usurp their throne, they'll be utterly loyal, and demand fidelity back. If you can treat them like royalty, and make them feel like it as well, they'll be the most enriching and romantic of partners.

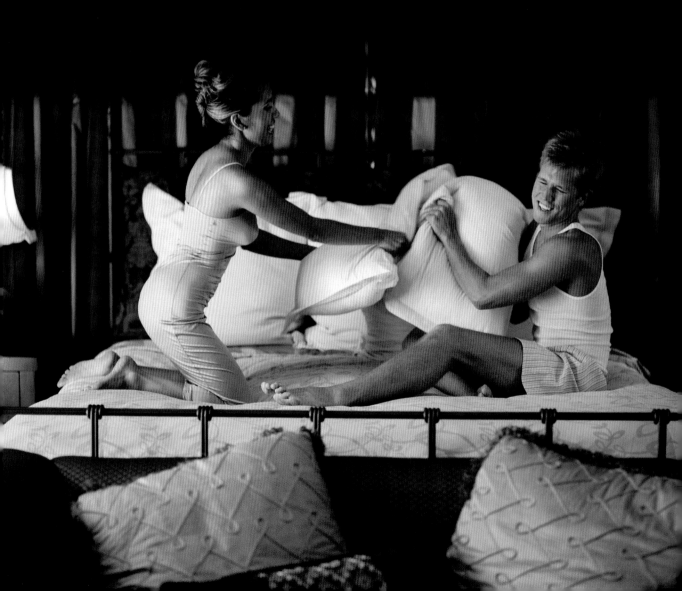

Show appreciation for all those little romantic gestures that Leo makes and you'll win yourself a magnanimous and warm-hearted companion for life. Leos do like long-term commitment, but they also need to feel they are the center of attention pretty much 24/7, otherwise the lion feels humiliated and sulks. Leos believe they are simply the best and deserve the best. Agree that they do, and seeing as your lion has chosen you, then that's you'll find you're included in a very glamorous lifestyle. Leos have an extraordinarily creative and romantic attitude to love and life, so if you share in that vision and never put them down, they'll crusade for your personal goals too and be utterly devoted.

LAZINESS
Most Leos want someone to trail around after them picking up the pieces. So if you're happy to do the housework, that's a

PRIDELESS LION

Leo loathes being anything less than number one in the relationship. So if you want Leo to dump you then it's a pretty painless and quick strategy. The trick is to show off in public, take over the limelight, and refuse to see eye to eye with your lion on anything. Before long he or she'll be eyeing up someone new! Never forget that, in the lion's universe, he or she is king or queen of the jungle. So if you act the part of the usurper then he or she'll soon be acting decisively to boot you out. If your world doesn't revolve around the lion, he or she'll be off to find another partner who knows it does!

> If you're ready to **stand back** and let your Leo **shine**, you can be a **long-term** consort to the **king or queen** of the jungle

exactly what he or she has got. Be prepared to take a backseat and let them shine, as they won't tolerate another diva in the relationship. If you can make it clear that the world revolves around them, then their worlds will revolve around you.

CRUSADER
Make it clear that you'll back them all the way regarding their careers or long-term goals, and bonus; if not, get a cleaner. Lions like to think they're the boss and will give you advice on how to do anything. So listen with eager attention, make a few bright suggestions, and Leo will immediately assume they were his or hers in the first place. This is not an easy sign to live with, but if you want spirit, excitement, and vitality in your life, then Leo's the most committed pussycat around.

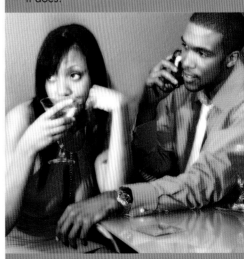

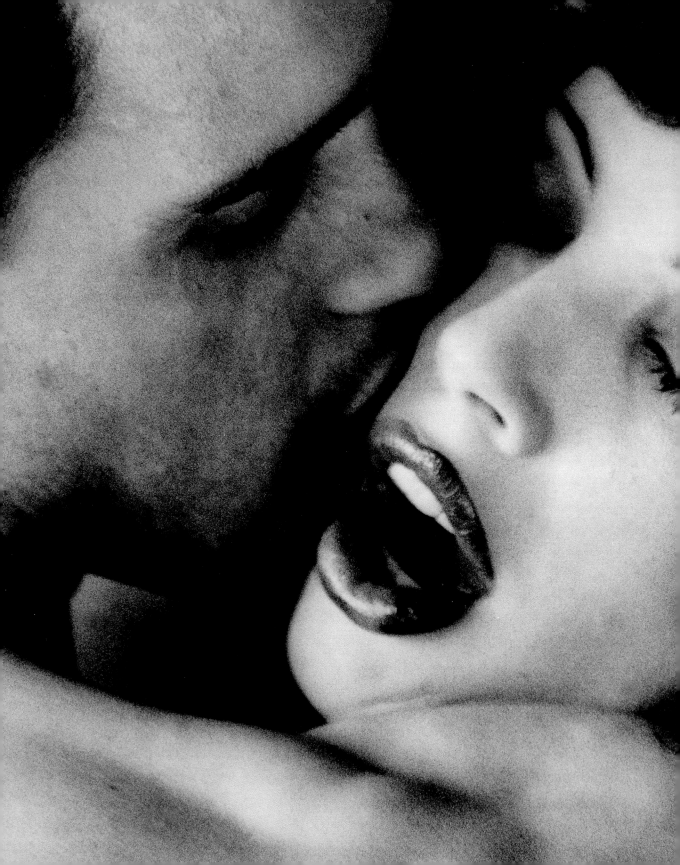

VIRGO

AUGUST 24 – SEPTEMBER 22

STAR STATS

Ruling planet MERCURY
Signature symbol THE VIRGIN
Metal BRONZE
Stone JADE
Color OCHER

Where to find Virgo Check out your local yoga class, health-food shops, and chic cafés. At parties, Virgo loves to help in the kitchen.

Hot date Romantic picnic in a secluded, back-to-nature spot.

Needs and desires Earthy, sensual, and secretly wicked, Virgo needs a dedicated partner and long-term commitment.

Top turn-on Being begged for sex, and then ripping each other's clothes off.

Sex positions ♀ Passion Fruit

♂ The Seesaw

Sex toy Kinky underwear.

Sex statistic 91 percent of Virgos are too shy to ask for what turns them on.

WHAT TO EXPECT WITH VIRGO

Virgos have a down-to-earth approach to sex and love and for them commitment means pretty much forever. Sensuous but discreet, Virgos aren't exactly fire and brimstone material in the bedroom, but they offer unrivaled dedication, affection, and long-term love.

Virgos are ruled by Mercury, the planet of communication and knowledge. That doesn't mean they just want to talk all night, but they do want to know all about you before they leap into bed, from your favorite book to the color of your pubic hair. And this sensual yet self-contained earth sign takes a while to warm up enough to check out if you're telling the truth about either.

On the other hand, talking about their sexual needs can be a little problematic because nine times out of ten Virgos hate appearing too demanding, and they'll hide behind a rather coy approach to intimacy. But they have an innate talent for mentally seducing you and physically arousing you before you've even realized it. Serene but hilarious, they are often chaotic about their body image behind the smooth, unruffled appearance. Seduce them with your immaculate looks and

dazzle them with your brainpower to turn on the heat.

MEETING OF MINDS

Virgos can be slow to get down to the nitty gritty. Renowned for their belief in sex manuals and skill in all aspects of lovemaking, they make sexual passion into a craft. However, they are very

protective and private about their innermost emotions and rarely let on how they feel about you even once you think you know them intimately—you never really will. Virgos are, however, the most interesting, witty, kind, and sensitive of lovers, but they need a relationship to be a true merger of minds.

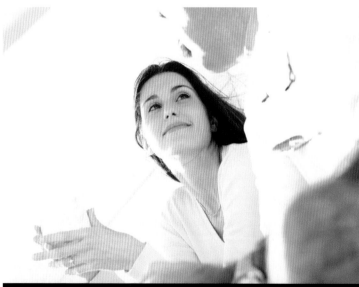

CONVERSATION LOVER Communicative Virgos are dazzled by your every word, as long as it's witty or intelligent!

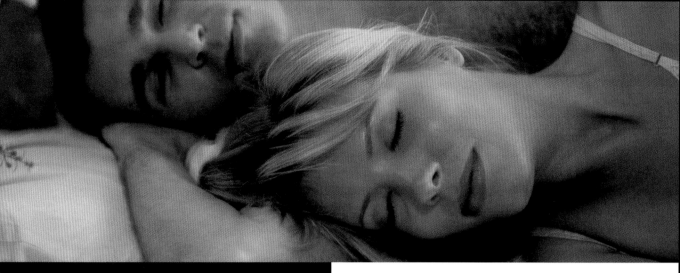

THE VIRGO MAN

Just because he's charming, well-dressed, and prefers a sensible lifestyle to wild partying, it doesn't mean that he's a bore in bed. Far from it. He's often the secret super-stud of the zodiac. Mr. Virgo has an earthy sex drive and is acutely sensitive, so he's often instinctively aware of your erogenous zones before you are. His body is his temple, and he won't mess around with anyone who won't appreciate his immaculate taste, penis size, technique, and style. Although he may take a while to let his barriers down, when he warms up he's hotter than hot, and more rampant than sometimes he admits to. And his performance? Well, it may be as sleek and sophisticated as he is, but then practice makes perfect, so it's usually orgasmically breathtaking too. Devoting a little time to getting to know him will definitely pay dividends!

THE VIRGO WOMAN

No silly games for this serene, self-possessed sensualist, no emotional angst, just what you see is what you get, and she usually wants to get it all the time. Real love takes time though: sex is a serious

> She's **slow** to open up, and likes to **keep** her sensual **mystique**

business and she expects any man to be as committed as she is. She makes dates as though they were business lunches and she makes love as if it was always the first time for her. She wants a reliable and communicative love relationship.

VIRGO IN A NUTSHELL

KEYWORDS Selective; dedicated; self-effacing; monogamous; sensual; intellectual; self-righteous; body-conscious; self-contained; communicative

LIKES Clean linen, socks, and a spotless bathroom; intelligent conversation; being pampered; honesty

DISLIKES Emotional scenes; ignorance; disorder; dirty fingernails

TRACKING DOWN YOUR VIRGO

Virgo is generally a self-contained, private sort of person, so you're not likely to bump into one on the dance floor or taking center stage at the bar. Intellectual but health-conscious, they like to keep fit and stick to the same routine, whether at the gym, in the office, or surfing the Internet for interesting facts and figures.

This mutable earth sign is also considered to be a bit of a nit-picker, so you often find them working in an environment where their critical skills can be put to use. Guided by their mercurial done, well-researched and double-checked for flaws. They assess information critically and make sure that everyone around them knows exactly what they're doing and, more importantly,

Virgos are very **aware** of their **spiritual** and bodily **health**, so the **serenity** of a spa is a good place to find this **private** sign

minds, their wide knowledge is earthed into practical, workable results. Virgos can edit anything, whether ideas, speeches, books, films, or your laundry. With a natural talent for getting the message across, they iron out other people's mistakes with flair and sophistication. With such high standards, people in more powerful positions intuitively know that Virgos get the job

why. There are some Virgos who make a living out of writing computer programs, which means they tend to stay out of the limelight, but you'll spot them in chic cafés with a laptop on the table.

HEALTH-CONSCIOUS
A little obsessed with the state of their health, Virgos are very conscious of their bodies and

image and are renowned for being squeaky clean. They like to work out, get fit, or go on fad diets, and they're rigorous about standards of food and hygiene. Punctuality is important to them because it means that they can control their lives. You'll find them in the same place every day at the same time. Check out your local health-food shop or delicatessen, the gym, sushi bar, or beneath a station clock (look out for the ones checking their watches while they are waiting impatiently for the train).

EDUCATION

Virgos adore learning and acquiring knowledge, and they often become eternal students or specialist teachers. Evening classes were invented for Virgo, and colleges, libraries, and bookstores are full of this dedicated, discriminating earth sign feeding on knowledge.

PLACES TO LOOK

SPAS AND HEALTH FARMS
Health-conscious Virgos favor a weekend break with like-minded people. They're usually the ones doing a headstand in the yoga class before anyone else.

BEAUTY COUNTER
Virgos are obsessed with cleanliness, body odors, and face creams. They'll pile up a shopping basket with the best beauty products, male or female.

LIBRARY OR BOOKSHOP
Very knowledgeable people need books to match. So head for the reference shelves or history section rather than the popular thrillers.

GARDEN
Like the other earth signs, Virgo has green fingers, and loves the back-to-nature vibe, puttering in a garden and growing vegetables.

VIRGO TOP TEN CAREERS

1 Literary agent
2 Secretary
3 Civil servant
4 Computer programmer
5 Copy editor
6 Critic
7 Dentist/Dental hygienist
8 Dietician
9 Healer
10 Pharmacist

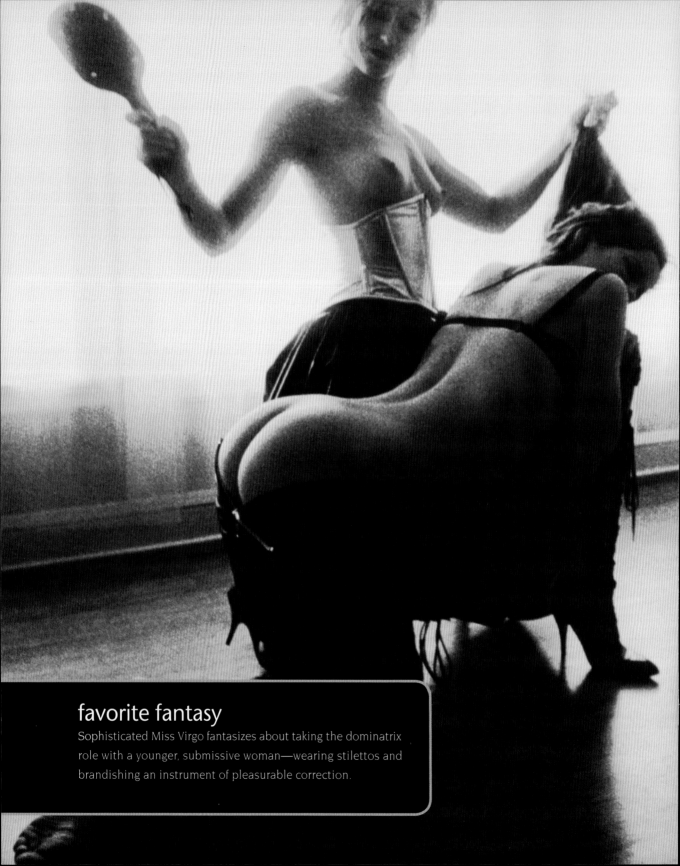

favorite fantasy

Sophisticated Miss Virgo fantasizes about taking the dominatrix role with a younger, submissive woman—wearing stilettos and brandishing an instrument of pleasurable correction.

WHAT WORKS FOR HER

This serene, classy woman needs a lover who respects her independence, privacy, and, above all, her sexual sophistication. For all her cool exterior, Miss Efficiency is one sensual woman under the bedcovers. Close up, she's dedicated and giving, and sensitive and refined in the art of lovemaking.

Virgo is, in fact, almost "virginal" in the way she approaches sex. Innocently seductive and rather cautious, she won't be up for one-night stands and expects a certain amount of dating protocol before heading for the bedroom. It takes a long time for a Virgo to feel confident about her own sexual needs. But if she knows what turns you on and you know just what turns her on then she'll abandon herself to spontaneous sensuous passion. Secretly, she's quite an authority on sex: the more knowledge she acquires, whether she reads about it,

> ## Miss Virgo is squeaky clean in body but wicked in bed

dreams about it, or simply does it, the more of a sex goddess she is.

LADY LOVE

Without doubt, Virgo's earthy sensuality comes to life once she can trust you and knows that you won't use her or make a fool of her. She's usually attracted to fitness fanatics who care about their bodies, as well as to sleek, silent men. As long as you know the difference between a clitoris and cunnilingus, are fascinated by her mind as well as her body, and have a passion for massage, you'll both experience mind-blowing sex. Sexually, you've got to know the ropes, be the perfect gentleman, and remember to discreetly place your underwear out of view of the bed.

HOW TO MAKE HER HORNY

The focal point of the Virgo woman's sexual energy flow is located at her navel, extending downward toward her pubis. She'll experience a powerful thrill if you brush your hand over this region while you are both still fully clothed. When you get to the naked stage, gently run your fingers up and down this sensitive astro-erogenous area first,

then softly lick and suck the skin around her navel, dabbling your tongue into the crevice. Don't rush or skimp on foreplay because she takes a long time to relax and lose her inhibitions. The slower and sexier the build-up is, the more your icy Virgo will respond by thawing her defenses and letting you in. To finish off, draw circles and spirals across her lower belly with your fingers, followed by your tongue. Take it from there!

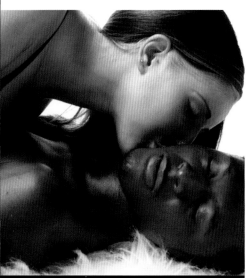

ULTIMATE SENSUALIST Once she trusts you and loses her inhibitions, Miss Virgo will adore taking charge and playing up to the role of the vampish dominatrix.

TANTALIZING

Cultivated and refined, the virgin of the zodiac likes gentle caresses and light teasing of lips and tongue. Sexual pleasure must be a mysterious ritual of arousal and subtle, classy foreplay. Elegant and delightful, she's the goddess of technique and earthy stimulation. Acutely sensitive to the touch, fragrance, and taste of your body, she wants to give rather than take. It can take her a long time to climax because she hates not being in control of her body or feelings, but when she does orgasm she's utterly abandoned. She often resists for as long as she can, or at least until she's persuaded herself that she's ready.

SOPHISTICATED

This elegant, classy lady conveys a deep exotic quality. She likes timing her orgasms to coincide with yours, but she also enjoys submissive sex and then flipping roles and dominating you when you least expect it. The Virgo woman also has a secret craving for sex toys, erotic literature, and mutual masturbation.

UP CLOSE AND PERSONAL

Miss Virgo's fear of disorder extends to her boudoir antics too. And until she's ready to respond to a surge of orgasmic energy, she prefers to start off with an up-close and basic sex position. Languid arousal and a lover with finesse who responds to her earthy sensuality is what the Virgo woman really craves. That's why the Passion Fruit is the perfect sex position for her. It aligns perfectly with her need for emotional intimacy, enabling her to enjoy a sensual and sophisticated experience. Not only does it let her take control of the first moments but it also allows her to yield when she's ready, caressing herself as you support her, lingering in the rhythm so that you gain total control. As she gets turned on by sharing the pleasure, her final orgasmic peak relies on

PASSION FRUIT

Try the Passion Fruit position first. The face-to-face intimacy allows her to watch your reactions and adjust her rhythm so you climax together. Her energy resonates to the same sexual energy flow as the other earth signs, so she'll also love the Mission Accomplished (see pages 40–41) and Orchid (see pages 184–85) positions. For this fruity starter, you sit on the edge of the bed with your feet on the ground.

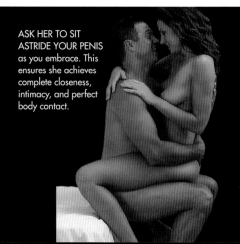

ASK HER TO SIT ASTRIDE YOUR PENIS as you embrace. This ensures she achieves complete closeness, intimacy, and perfect body contact.

HER TOP TURNOFFS

SHABBY CLOTHES
She really does loathe untidiness. So if you want to score brownie points with your immaculate outfit, don't forget to wear designer underwear too.

FAST AND FURIOUS
Hard, penetrative intercourse isn't so cool for her as lengthy oral sex: she needs time to get fully aroused.

IDIOTS
Quite honestly, if you don't have a brain to match hers, then forget it. She's needs a smart, fit man, not a thickhead.

LAZINESS
If you can't be bothered to work at your ambitions or body image, then she won't want to play with you either. Dedication matters to this classy woman!

knowing that she can trust you to come too.

SQUEAKY CLEAN
Once she feels you're worthy of her stylish attention, your sensitive touch and the quality of the surroundings are big erotic triggers. Make love on fine cotton sheets or on fake furs before a log fire. Her favorite sexual trigger is watching you when you orgasm, and she also adores getting wet and steamy. Lather her up in the shower and then take the showerhead and ask her to point it first on your penis and then on her clitoris. Rub your penis between her buttocks while she masturbates. Then make love between soft white towels while you're still both wet.

DIRTY TALK
Virgos are often very shy about revealing their erotic fantasies,

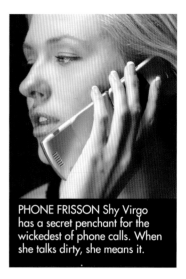

PHONE FRISSON Shy Virgo has a secret penchant for the wickedest of phone calls. When she talks dirty, she means it.

early on in the relationship, anyway. But once she starts to trust you, she's slowly aroused by whispering her wickedest thoughts in your ear and hearing yours in return. Mercury-ruled, Virgo will discuss sex in clinical detail as though it's a long list of ingredients for a soufflé, but she's also the secret diva of dirty talk, wicked whispers, text messages, and erotic phone calls.

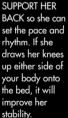

SUPPORT HER BACK so she can set the pace and rhythm. If she draws her knees up either side of your body onto the bed, it will improve her stability.

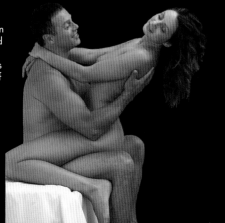

WHEN YOU ARE BOTH READY TO CLIMAX, cup her buttocks and gather her toward you for sensational closeness. The feeling of being supported enables her to abandon herself to pleasure.

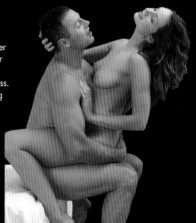

WHAT WORKS FOR HIM

Slick and sophisticated, Mr. Virgo is one of the most decent and down-to-earth signs. His polished performance is timed to perfection, and he really does care what's going on in your mind as well as between your legs. A true gentleman he may be, but don't underestimate his passionate libido.

A conventional lover, Mr. Virgo likes to stick to the rules of seduction. This means he's in control of the game and can decide whether he wants to get involved with you before it gets too messy and out of his hands (disorder is his worst nightmare). Virgo believes in one step at a time, whether you're heading to the bedroom or the altar. And he rather likes it if you seduce him in chronological order. This sensual and incredibly useful man is mostly concerned about what comes out of your mouth. It gives him many clues about what is going on in your head, which is as important to him as the curvature of your breasts or the line of your buttocks (which are equal in his mind, although he'll probably never admit it).

On a first date, resort to age-old traditions of etiquette and let him open the door for you. Once he's convinced you're also extremely knowledgeable, then the sexier pursuits can begin. Sensual, private, and highly erotic, Mr. Virgo does take his time. So if you're impatient or want to leap into the flames of torrid passion, think again.

ICEBOX

Whether he likes to admit it or not, sexual arousal involves feelings that are alien to his cool, slick image. Things like love and anger or jealousy and sentimentality are treated more like bits of clutter to be kept hidden under the laundry basket, thanks very much. That's when he takes on the persona of "Mr. Textbook Technique" because he'd rather not think about wild passions, libidos, and sex drives which are, after all, very animal, very mysterious, and mean he's not in control of his senses.

HOW TO MAKE HIM HORNY

Mr. Virgo is a touchy-feely man, but he likes foreplay to be pretty straightforward and predictable, so don't go for any surprises. Focus on the area around his navel and lower belly: that rather fine line that goes down to his groin is one of his most sensitive turn-on down the sex-line and run them nimbly across to his thighs without touching his penis. Follow through exactly the same format with your tongue around this potent astro-erogeneous zone and then kiss the inside of his thighs and he'll be in Virgo heaven. Don't forget that your mind is a big turn-on for the Virgo man as well, so he'll adore it if you add in some sexy

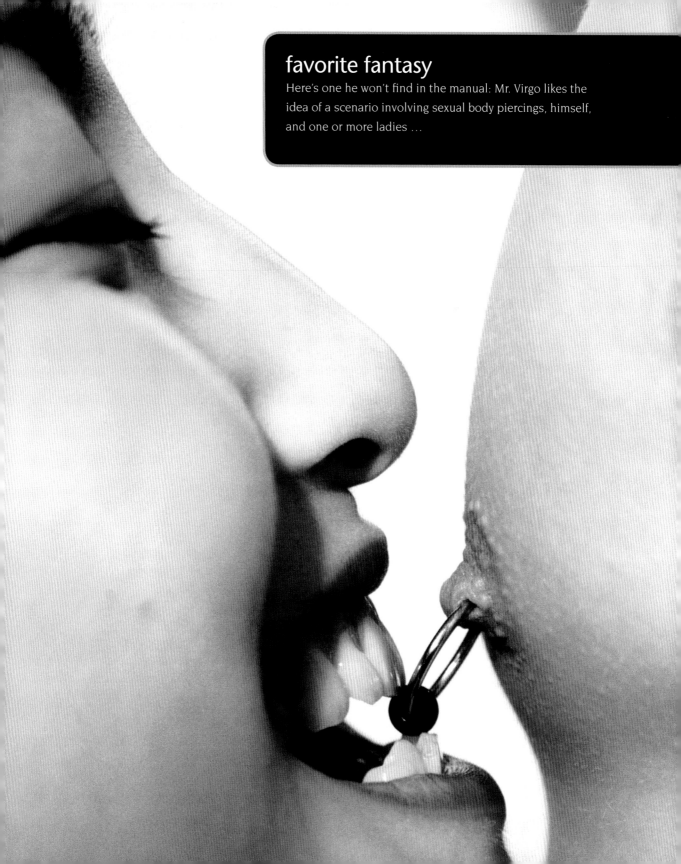

favorite fantasy

Here's one he won't find in the manual: Mr. Virgo likes the idea of a scenario involving sexual body piercings, himself, and one or more ladies ...

PERFECTION AND PRIVACY

Remember, the sexiest thing about you—apart from your perfect body—is your mind. He's turned on by intellectual chit-chat along with initial physical contact, because it makes him feel in control of his senses rather than totally out of them! Mr. Virgo hates emotional scenes and drama queens. He's not exactly the exhibitionist kind and will totally shun any physical contact in public, such as obvious signs of teasing or fondling beneath the restaurant table. But in private his technique and mastery are unparalleled.

CHAMPAGNE ON ICE

When young, he may seem a little obsessed with routine sex. It's not that he's boring, but just trying to get it absolutely right. Once he's mastered a technique then he'll move on to something new. And once he's mastered you, take care, because for all his apparent loyalty, fidelity, and earthy reliability, he's ruled by flighty Mercury and is changeable and restless. However, as Mr. Virgo matures, he becomes less obsessed with perfecting the art of sex and more fascinated by your mind. Emotions and sexual abandon? Well, those are still fearful things to him. Like all earth signs, he's happy with his physical prowess but isn't happy to be controlled by his sex drive.

Once you get to know Mr. Virgo a bit better, you'll be pleased to hear that his biggest turn-ons are sensual. White linen, champagne on ice, expensive perfumes, and a fresh, clean, and feminine body. He adores playing dominant one minute, the next a sexual voyeur. Surprise him (once you get to

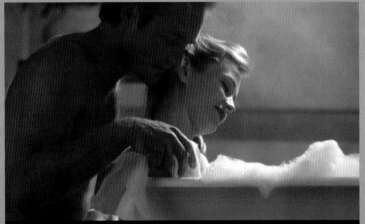

WET DREAMS Let Mr. Virgo help out in the bathtub. He'll be turned on by soaping everything from your breasts to your toes.

THE SEESAW

He may be the cool, technical perfectionist of the zodiac, but he does require equality and physical closeness in the bedroom. One of his favorite starting points is to begin both sitting facing one another, your legs hooked over his arms. From this position you can move freely through the Seesaw sequence to lying down or man-on-top positions, changing the sexual power dynamic.

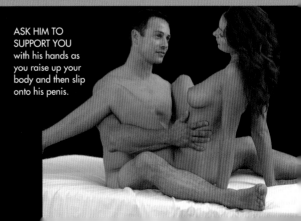

ASK HIM TO SUPPORT YOU with his hands as you raise up your body and then slip onto his penis.

know him, he's up for unpredictability; after all, it keeps him on his toes) when he visits and be in the bath or shower and invite him to join you. Ask him to lick your fingers while you masturbate yourself with them. Then give him oral sex while you buzz of wearing clothes while you're both masturbating, then stripping each other naked and getting really close with *soixante-neuf*, one of his favorite oral sex positions. Remember, he likes perfecting techniques, so let him practice as long as he likes;

> The Virgo man **appreciates** that **sex is an art** and goes to great lengths to **perfect** his technique

slide your fingers between his lips. Wet your nipples with champagne and let him lick it off.

PRACTICE MAKES PERFECT

Mr. Virgo adores alternating between submissive and dominating positions, so be prepared to change roles and take the initiative. He loves the let him check the sex manual beside the bed and let him follow the instructions: he'll be the ultimate master of pure, seductive lovemaking, and the best lover around for giving you multiple orgasms. When you've taken all the necessary steps to mate for life, he's up for a lot more experimentation.

HIS TOP TURNOFFS

WILDCATS
Virgo hates anything that doesn't fit into his routine, so if you're a wildcat, put your claws away. He won't play.

DIRT
He may have a dirty mind in the bedroom, but he loathes other kinds of filth. BO, smelly breath, and dirty fingernails are his major turnoffs.

SOCIAL EMBARRASSMENT
He won't kiss you in public. He's terrified of being ruled by those ghastly "animal passions" or, worse still, an erection.

SOGGY TISSUES
Emotional stuff puts Virgo in a panic, and sessions where emotions get splattered around turn him into a nervous wreck.

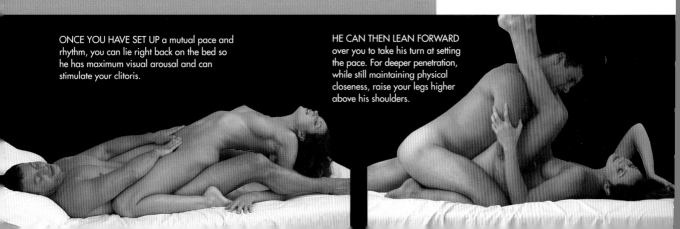

ONCE YOU HAVE SET UP a mutual pace and rhythm, you can lie right back on the bed so he has maximum visual arousal and can stimulate your clitoris.

HE CAN THEN LEAN FORWARD over you to take his turn at setting the pace. For deeper penetration, while still maintaining physical closeness, raise your legs higher above his shoulders.

IS THIS THE ONE?

Virgos seek a balance between the passion they secretly desire and the routine that makes them feel safe. If you're looking for a technically efficient, sensual, and wise lover, and can bring out a Virgo's hidden fire, you'll never be bored.

ARIES AND VIRGO

Definitely an attraction of very different types, and could be seriously romantic and steamy if Virgo accepts Aries' extrovert needs and Aries understands Virgo's more private ones. A fine working relationship if you keep your independence.

TAURUS AND VIRGO

Once you realize that you share a love of nature, as well as a very sensual and sexy rapport, there's very little to keep you apart. A warm, trusting relationship. Problems arise if Virgo's on a health kick and decides the bull's too self-indulgent.

GEMINI AND VIRGO

Both ruled by Mercury, but will be an instant attraction or an instant repulsion. Virgo thinks that Gemini is intellectually inferior and is liable to nag the twins, so Gemini may get silently resentful. Not easy, but very sexy.

CANCER AND VIRGO

Virgo feels very safe in Cancer's needy arms, but the crab's sensitive, unpredictable moods can be too chaotic for Virgo's cool and ordered approach to life. An enriching sexual rapport, but not easy long-term unless Virgos can be more open.

LEO AND VIRGO

Workable and creative, as you respect each other's different approach to life. But Virgo might begin to resent Leo's constant flamboyant antics in public, while Leo will get fed up with having to be punctual and organized.

VIRGO AND VIRGO

Mutual understanding of your weaknesses and virtues. But you probably won't bring to life either's passionate, wild side. Great for a working relationship, but lacking romance, and you are likely to be highly critical of each other.

Physical and mental **harmony**. However, Libra is far more **idealistic** than Virgo and could get disillusioned by Virgo's realism. And Libra's **perfectionist tendencies** will grate on Virgo. Good **long-term rapport** though.

LIBRA AND VIRGO

Virgos feel like they've been thrown in **at the deep end** with one very hungry beast, compelled into a **transformative** relationship. Scorpio likes to play **intellectual power games** with Virgo, but there's a distinct sexual attraction here.

SCORPIO AND VIRGO

Virgo must be ready to **follow** Sagittarius across mountains. Could prove to be a highly **exciting adventure** *à deux*, if Virgo can tolerate the archer's **unreliability** and Sagittarius can accept criticism. Very **dynamic**, but ultimately hard work.

SAGITTARIUS AND VIRGO

A wonderful **sexual rapport** that relies on a bond of **companionship**. Likely to be a serious long-lasting involvement. **Stability**, materialism, and work are important considerations for these signs for **long-term happiness**.

CAPRICORN AND VIRGO

A highly **unusual relationship** based on intellectual rapport. Aquarius is fascinated by Virgo's **sensible** streak, and Virgo by Aquarius' detached view of love and life. Great for **loving friendship**, but you might come to blows over money and sex.

AQUARIUS AND VIRGO

Natural opposites of the zodiac usually attract. You have tense then **teasing sexual moments**, totally insatiable and unstoppable. Arousal is **profound** and you develop a haunting **devotion** to one another. Unique and satisfying.

PISCES AND VIRGO

AND THE WINNER IS...

It's not easy to choose a winner, as Virgo needs to have both the practical, workable, intellectual rapport as well as the wilder, passionate type of relationship to feel really happy. However, the other earth signs, Taurus and Capricorn, are favorites for long-term stability. But for grand passion, romance, and a chance for Virgos to liberate themselves from the chains of fear and to play rather than always work, then Pisces comes out as the winner.

LONG-TERM LOVE WITH VIRGO

It's not that Virgos are seeking a paragon, but they do need to have a partner who makes sense and can hold their own in a discussion or debate on anything from world economics to why dildos are must-have saucy accessories. Virgos thrive in close, long-term partnerships with people who are also secret romantics like themselves.

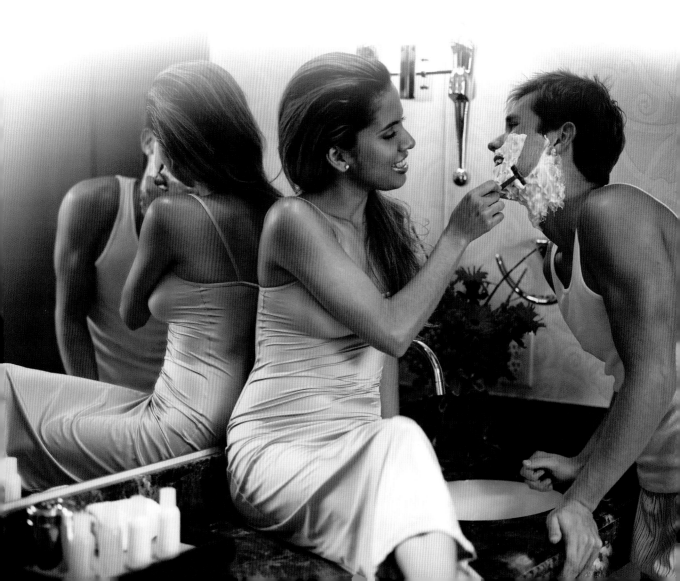

Feelings of real "love" take a long time to mature for Virgo, and they prefer partners who are organized, orderly, and mature. If you're up for scrubbing floors, painting everything white, and living a rather minimalist kind of lifestyle with zinc stoves, no pets, and high-tech gadgets on every wall, then Virgo is for you. Virgo wants delicacy, discretion, and discrimination in a partner, with a little bit of that healing

will be left in heaps, and their jeans piled up ready for ironing. Be one step ahead and tidy up before they do and they'll love you even more.

REAPING THE REWARDS

Virgos are very useful to have around in lots of ways. They know how things work, they will make love a sensual and rewarding experience, and once they feel they're in control of their lives then they're quite happy to

VIRGO-ING, GOING, GONE!

Virgo gets obsessed with routine and likes everything to be exactly in its place. And that includes you. So if you want to push your Virgo into getting rid of you, there's nothing more liable to drive him or her up the wall than being unreliable, both around the home and in your mind. Vacillate about whether or not you should do something, hold back from making decisions, change your routine for no apparent reason, and unleash your unpredictable side. You'll soon throw your collected Virgo off balance—and they'll throw you out.

> If you like **order** in your life as well and can **balance** out the Virgo **obsessive streak**, you could be an **ideal match**

fire in their sexual relationships. Be as dedicated to their strategic, organised way of life as they are, and you'll have a mate for life.

HOUSE PROUD

Virgos are either incredibly tidy or a total mess around the home. They call the latter, "organized chaos." And Virgos will insist they're the best cleaners around. But it's probably their socks or panties rather than yours that

ring the changes accordingly. And, believe it or not, there is a dreamy, sensitive soul behind that cool, unruffled, intellectual approach to life. So if you can offer trust, warmth, closeness and seduce them into the occasional chill-out time where your workaholic Virgo can flip to a playful spirit, this self-contained and magical realist will give you respect, intelligent thinking, and loyalty by the bucketload.

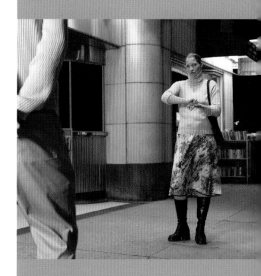

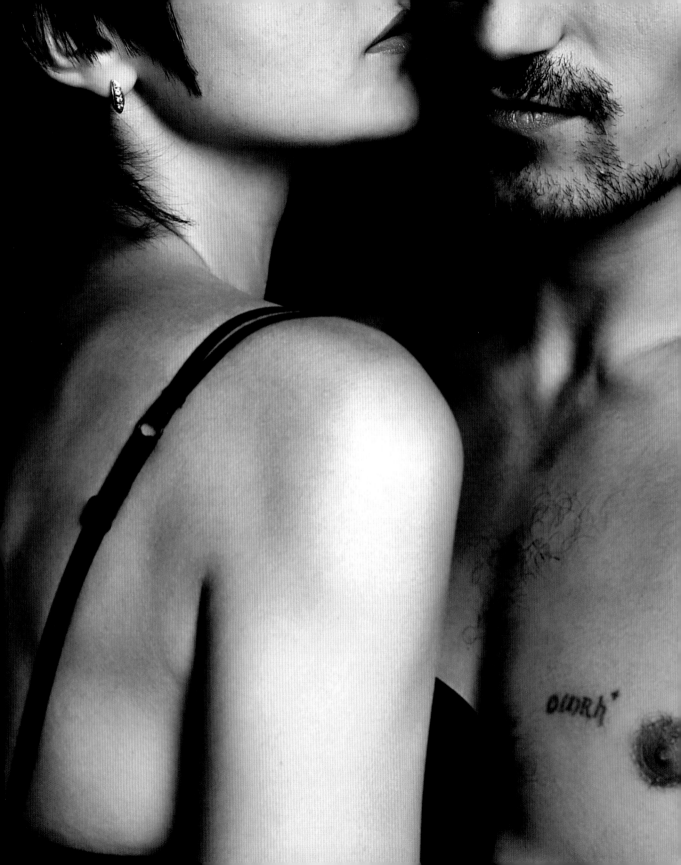

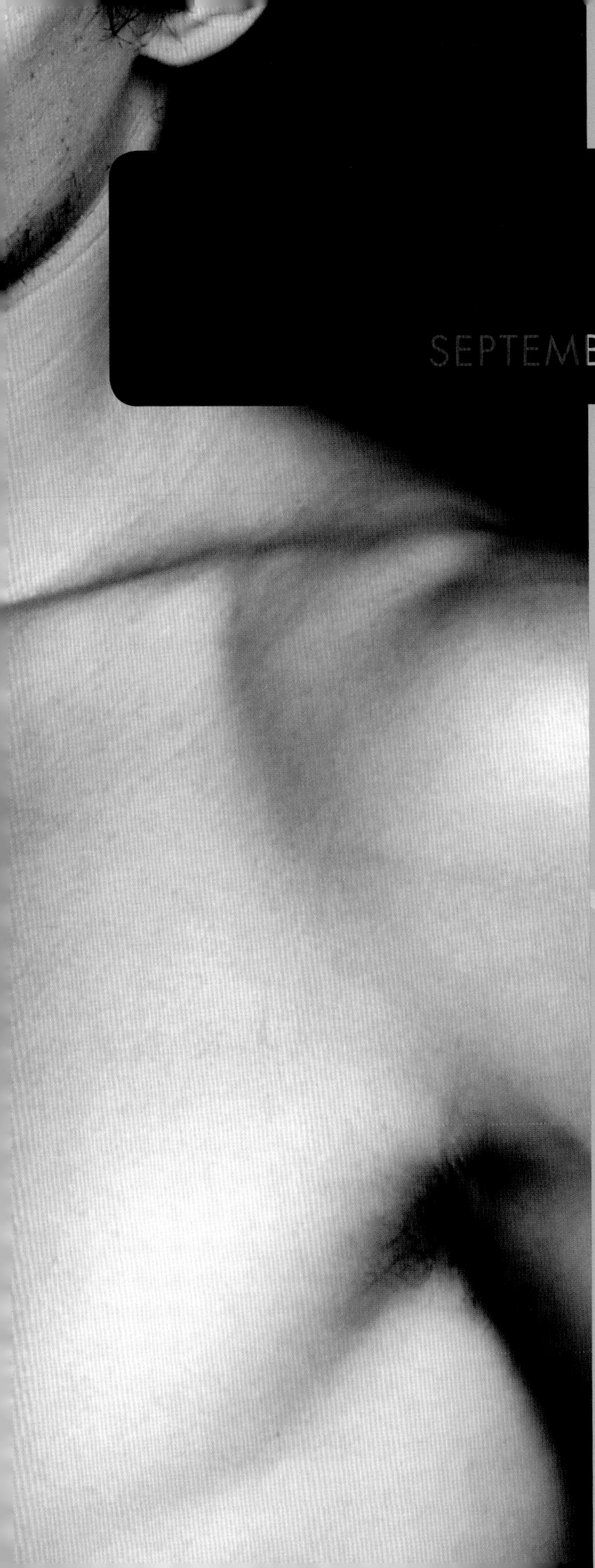

LIBRA

SEPTEMBER 23 — OCTOBER 23

STAR STATS

Ruling planet VENUS

Signature symbol THE SCALES

Metal COPPER

Stone CARNELIAN

Color BRIGHT GREEN

Where to find Libra Hanging out in art galleries, spas, and at all the best cocktail parties or soirées.

Hot date A candlelit dinner overlooking a beautiful view.

Needs and desires Aesthetic and charming, Libra is an utter idealist about love and sex and desperately seeks the perfect partner.

Top turn-on Secret oral sex in discreet public locations.

Sex positions ♀ Cherry Blossom
♂ Horseplay

Sex toy Fur love cuffs.

Sex statistic 79 percent of Librans can't say no to a fling.

Venus-ruled Libra is an air sign, and is one of the most charming, seductive, and idealistic of the zodiac signs. This utter romantic lives in a wafty cloud-cuckoo land about love and sex. Convinced they'll one day find the perfect partner, it's actually hard for anyone to live up to their divine vision.

Venus wasn't just the goddess of sex and earthly delights, she was also vain, idealistic, and concerned with geometrical beauty. Libra certainly lives up to this airy side of Venus's domain. The scales want the world to be in balance and they'll make sure it is by playing the role of charmer to secretly get what they want. Beauty is important to Librans, both yours and theirs. In fact, they can be so vain or insecure about their body image that they overdo the makeup or snazzy shoes and are often renowned socially for being the "brutes in Armani suits," both male and female.

DIPLOMATIC SERVICE

The diplomats of the zodiac are smooth, refined, and intellectual. They need an equal, so they're looking for taste, class, perfection and good looks. A well-designed house, a cool car, you name it: Libra desires aesthetically pleasing things. This is where Librans have the odd problem, for all their grace, pacifism and witty conversations: the earthy instincts of lust, sweating bodies and emotional passion just don't fit into their ideal vision of romance. That's why their charmingly seductive behavior when you first meet them—the romantic dinners, the candles, expensive perfume, gifts, and flirtatious remarks—is all part of a big game. What they're truly looking for isn't steamy passion and marathon penetrative sex all night, but the chance to linger under the stars and dream of what might be, to imagine a perfect sexual relationship with their dream lover rather than actually engage in the heat of the moment with a real, fallible partner.

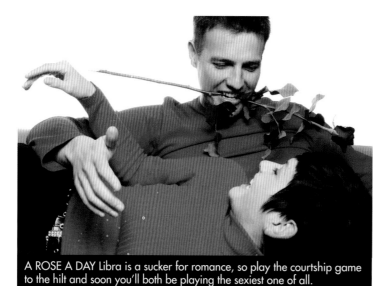

A ROSE A DAY Libra is a sucker for romance, so play the courtship game to the hilt and soon you'll both be playing the sexiest one of all.

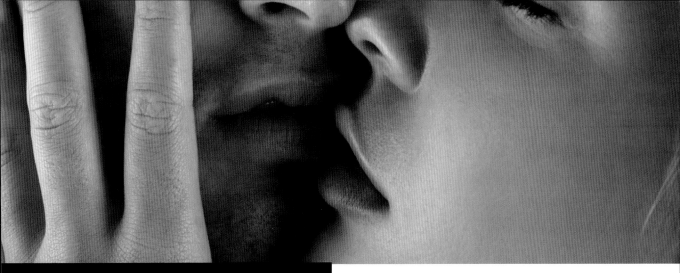

THE LIBRA MAN

Mr. Prince Charming falls in love with any aspect from your hair to eyes or smile if it lives up to his ideal image. He's a natural flirt and could sell saunas in a rainforest. In fact, he's pretty sure he's

> Mr. Libra is the ideal lover: he's polite and ready to please

Adonis and is on the lookout for romance and beauty wherever he goes. Socially correct, beautifully dressed, what you see is what you get. In bed you can expect a polished performance and the romantic interlocking of minds.

THE LIBRA WOMAN

She's charming. She's chatty, flirtatious, and fun to have around. She adores socializing and wants to talk about "us" and not "me." Yet this romantic princess of the zodiac is also intellectually driven to succeed. Miss Libra lives in her head, and all those ghastly things called emotions and feelings are repressed. Men can't help but swoon in her presence and admire her impeccable taste. Socially adept in all the arts of seduction, there's an air of femininity about her that women find threatening, and men find fascinating. But she's an approval seeker and finds it hard to say "no." She's so willing to please that she may not know what she wants herself. Libra believes that if someone fancies her then all she has to do is say "yes" and her dream will come true. Falling in love is easy for Libra because she loves the idea rather than the reality.

LIBRA IN A NUTSHELL

KEYWORDS Seductive; indecisive; sophisticated; idealistic; subtle; rational; paradoxical; compliant; manipulative

LIKES Compliments; romantic conversations; beautiful people; socializing

DISLIKES Arguments; emotional scenes; loneliness; heavy commitment; splitting up

TRACKING DOWN YOUR LIBRA

Librans are social animals. They adore partying at all the best places and are usually popular, so it's pretty easy to track them down. They prefer light-hearted chitchat with a crowd of people to staying at home, so get out to your local haunts and you're sure to bump into the charmer of the zodiac.

Easygoing and diplomatic, Librans thrive in an environment where everyone is an equal, or appears to be. If they have to muck in or muck out they'll do it just to show that they're

TIPPING THE BALANCE

Librans have a natural instinct for bringing people together and a knack for making sure fair is fair and all is above board. They make brilliant solicitors

Gregarious Librans are pretty **easy to find**, but it'll be more difficult to **make your mark**

everyone's friend. With an amazing visual and aesthetic talent, they will be a success in the world of fashion, beauty, design, or anything that is to do with taste. Librans are usually beautifully packaged articles themselves and tend to create an atmosphere of perfection around them. This gives them the effortless power to charm and persuade the opposite sex to their way of doing things in a very subtle way.

and bankers, but you're more likely to find Librans beautifying the world and the people in it by working in a glamorous environment or a profession where they receive approval for their diplomatic skills.

PARTY ANIMAL

Socially adept, Librans like to be liked. So they usually head for the social circle of the opposite sex (to test their seductive skills) rather than the singles' bar. You'll find Libran women prefer to hang out with a group of intellectually bright men, and Libran men like to hold forth surrounded by adoring females. At any party, Libra is instantly recognizable by being the most popular person there. Or, if new to the social scene, they'll be the ones who borrow the wine bottle and share it in an attempt to get to know everyone they come across.

ART LOVERS

Venus-ruled Libra loves art in many forms, from modern to classical, sculpture to holograms. The chances are they'll be visiting a gallery or running it, working behind the scenes in the theater, slapping makeup on film stars, or working on their body image at a local health spa or chic holiday resort. They're suckers for a little fame and fortune too, so you'll often spot them in posh restaurants and exclusive clubs.

PLACES TO LOOK

ELITE CLUBS AND RESTAURANTS
It's not so much the food as the ambience, style, and social cachet. The scales can't bear to be seen anywhere less than perfect.

HAIRDRESSERS
Librans are extravagant when it comes to taking care of their looks, and why not? They want to be beautiful and their hair is always in top-notch condition.

WEDDINGS
Librans' romantic streak lures them to wedding parties. They have airy visions of happily-ever-after marriages, and idealize the whole white wedding trip.

FLORISTS
Librans adore fresh-cut flowers. If they're not buying a bunch of lilies for their home, they'll be hoping to bump into another orchid lover.

LIBRA TOP TEN CAREERS

1 Makeup artist/Beauty therapist
2 Hairdresser
3 Model
4 Art dealer
5 Wedding organizer
6 Graphic designer
7 Interior designer
8 Marriage counsellor
9 Diplomat
10 Lawyer/Business consultant

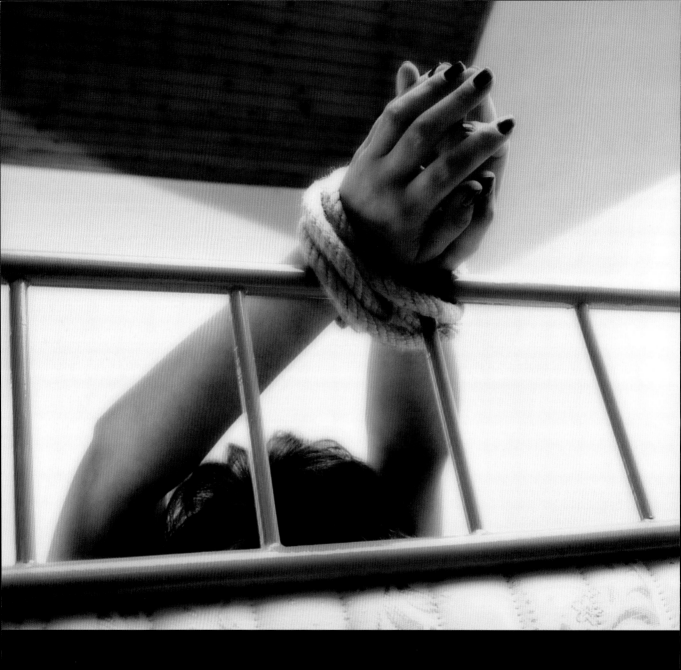

favorite fantasy

Miss Libra's romantic imagination secretly thrills to the idea
of being held captive and tied to a bed in a high tower where
a beautiful youth ravishes her each night.

WHAT WORKS FOR HER

A talent for harmonious relationships and her feminine beauty and witty conversations are the things that make the Libra woman a beautiful catch. She's ultimately trying to find the perfect balance both in and out of bed, and keep her life running smoothly on an even keel.

Attracted to much older, younger, or culturally different men, she's forever trying to prove opposites attract and can live in harmony as well. Seeking a perfect sex life to match isn't easy though. Libra often falls in love with a face, a body, a mood, a glance and then finds out later that all isn't quite as dreamy as she thought. That's why she often gets disillusioned when sex starts to complicate her airy ideal of romance.

BEAUTIFUL SEX
Seductive and utterly feminine, it's the actual chase (albeit a

> Sex must be a **beautiful** and **beautifying** experience, one that **eroticizes** her **mind** first and her **body** second

rather subtle one) that vitalizes her libido. Romance is one of her biggest turn-ons and she needs to passively dominate in order to maximize her erotic impulse. In fact, when she's in control and on top, she's the diva of orgasmic bliss. But it's a romantic,

knight-in-shining-armor approach that unleashes her sexual appetite. It's not lush and earthy like Taurus or intense and steamy like Scorpio. Her partner must be polished but passionate, strong but gentle, but also be prepared to give her lots of personal space.

HOW TO MAKE HER HORNY

Romance is the one thing that she really craves. And you'd better make sure that you supply the ambience too. Light some candles or dim the lights, plump up the cushions, and set the scene as though you were creating a movie. Stroke her gently all over with a beautiful ostrich feather while she runs her fingers over your immaculate body. It's the sight

of you together naked in the flickering candlelight that will do more to make this romantic princess horny than any textbook technique. Follow up with gentle caresses along the outside of her thighs and up across her buttocks to really drive her wild with anticipation. Her astro-erogeneous zone is centered around the lower spine and upper thigh region, so a little attention in this area is sure to get the scales tipped in your favor.

SENSITIVITY

The Libran woman is sensitive to every gesture and needs delicate and lengthy foreplay mixed with erotic talk and anticipation of what's to come. A table for two at your favorite restaurant, soft music, a bottle of champagne, and a tranquil environment satisfy her desire for romantic lovemaking and enable her to lose any inhibitions. Turn the lights down low, though: for all her fabulous clothes, hair, and perfume, she has low sexual self-esteem and can be shy.

VISUAL AROUSAL

Libra's sexual expression is subtly seductive. She has the power of both coy arousal and unawakened passion. Your face, body, and sexual prowess are the perfect ingredients to allow her mind to work in tandem with her physical arousal. The epicenter

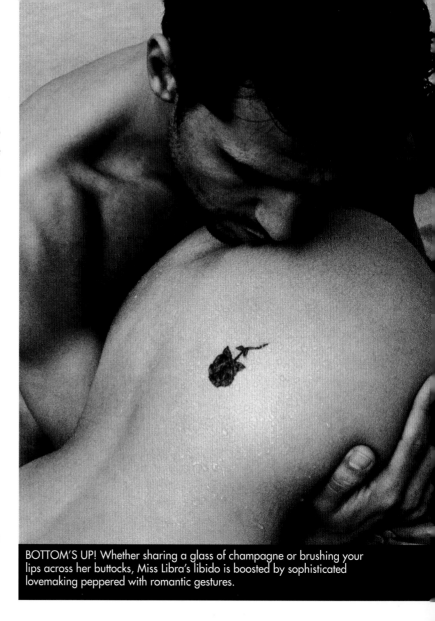

BOTTOM'S UP! Whether sharing a glass of champagne or brushing your lips across her buttocks, Miss Libra's libido is boosted by sophisticated lovemaking peppered with romantic gestures.

CHERRY BLOSSOM

When it comes to sex positions, the Libran woman craves a beautifully romantic experience, which is why the Cherry Blossom is perfect. This position enables her be at her most captivating and seductive and yet retain tenderness and sexual warmth. The visual power of your erection stimulates her sexual energy flow. Slow thrusts will lead to the most luscious and bonding of mutual orgasms.

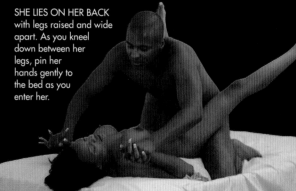

SHE LIES ON HER BACK with legs raised and wide apart. As you kneel down between her legs, pin her hands gently to the bed as you enter her.

HER TOP TURNOFFS

ONE-NIGHT SHAG
Libra can be promiscuous, but she believes lust is about in-loveness, so never ask her for a "quick shag": making love is making love.

SWEAT AND TEARS
She loathes smelly feet, sweaty armpits, and emotional wrecks.

POSSESSIVE ATTITUDES
If there's one thing Libra can't bear, it's being jealously guarded. She needs her space to socialize and flirt, so grin and bear it.

LOUD-MOUTHS AND UGLY DUCKLINGS
Visually, you've got to be a bit of a catch, but what comes out of your mouth and is in your head is just as important. So make sure that you're as refined in speech and thought as you are in looks.

of her sexual energy flow begins at the base of her spine and is a powerful libido boosting point. Tongue, lick, or caress her from the cleft of her buttocks up as far as the beginning of her spine, and use long sweeping movements of hand, lips, mouth, or penis for sizzling arousal.

ROMANTIC
When it comes to sex, Libra craves a beautifully romantic experience, which is why the Cherry Blossom position is perfect for her. Libra likes to maintain visual contact, so you can move from this position to the Genie Rub (see pages 58–59) or Maverick (see pages 202–203) positions: this sign resonates to the same sexual energy flow as the other air signs, Gemini and Aquarius. Make sure you keep the erotic communication flowing as well as the physical

contact between you, as this is a real turn-on for her.

SUBMISSIVELY DOMINANT
Much as she adores submitting, she does so by leading you on to do what she wants while you believe you're in charge of the show! The Libra lady loves to please, which means she's actually pleasing herself. She adores fantasy sex, pretending she's a virgin being initiated on your altar of pleasure or playing the houri or the mistress of a Roman emperor. Gentle bondage turns her on too, so lightly bind her wrists behind her back with a silk scarf and run your tongue across her belly down to her clitoris. Then lie in submissive position yourself and let her, still bound at the wrists, sit astride you and rub her clitoris against the tip of your penis. She'll adore playing both roles!

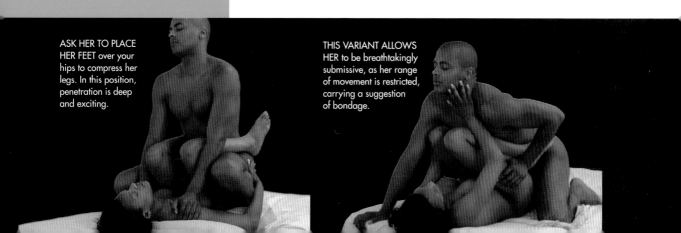

ASK HER TO PLACE HER FEET over your hips to compress her legs. In this position, penetration is deep and exciting.

THIS VARIANT ALLOWS HER to be breathtakingly submissive, as her range of movement is restricted, carrying a suggestion of bondage.

WHAT WORKS FOR HIM

Well, it has to be said that Mr. Libra is the ultimate Don Juan of the zodiac. Really, you can't go wrong with him. He's perfectly charming, utterly sexy, always well-dressed and preened, and is funny and graceful. And underneath that idealistic charmer lurks a sex drive matched by few.

> Noncommittal and **airy**, Mr. Libra adds up to one **sophisticated** but **paradoxical** package

He is a romantic, and because he lives in such an idealistic head, he doesn't quite realize that sex is also about bodily secretions, harsh morning light, and the odd squelch. But stay looking as good as him, and you'll find he'll give you the kind of sex you want all night and all day. He wants to please you, so please yourself!

ROMANTIC SEX-GOD

Find any excuse to bend down on a first date. A hint of cleavage or a glimpse of your sexy bra will stir him into action. However, this ideal *homme* isn't quite what he seems on first encounter. He needs to keep his romantic vision of you, so avoid mud-packs, panties lying around, and, if you're all noise when you climax, think about whether this is the man for you: he prefers breathless whispers in his ear.

VANISHING ACT

He is a perfectionist, and he may put up with the Tampax box and God-knows-what around his love nest while he's wooing you, but not for long. Be beautiful, in bed and out of it, or you'll find he's the incredible vanishing man. Sweaty, torrid sex isn't his game, nor is emotional power-tripping, but if you're all sweetness and light, he'll take you to the stars.

HOW TO MAKE HIM HORNY

Mr. Libra is rather lazy in the foreplay department. In fact, he's usually up for you doing all the work while he sits back and luxuriates in being turned on. Basically whatever pleases you, pleases him: it's his kind of passive way of taking control. Stay fully dressed, or half-dressed in your sexiest lingerie, and keep the lights down low (otherwise he'll get distracted by the clutter in the room or the spot on your chin). His lower spine and upper thighs are his prime astro-erogenous zones. Ask him to lie on his front—he'll soon be writhing against the bed linen if you use gentle massage-like pressure from your fingers around the small of his back. Follow on by stroking his outer thighs, then his inner ones without going anywhere near his penis. By now even the most indolent Libran should be standing at attention

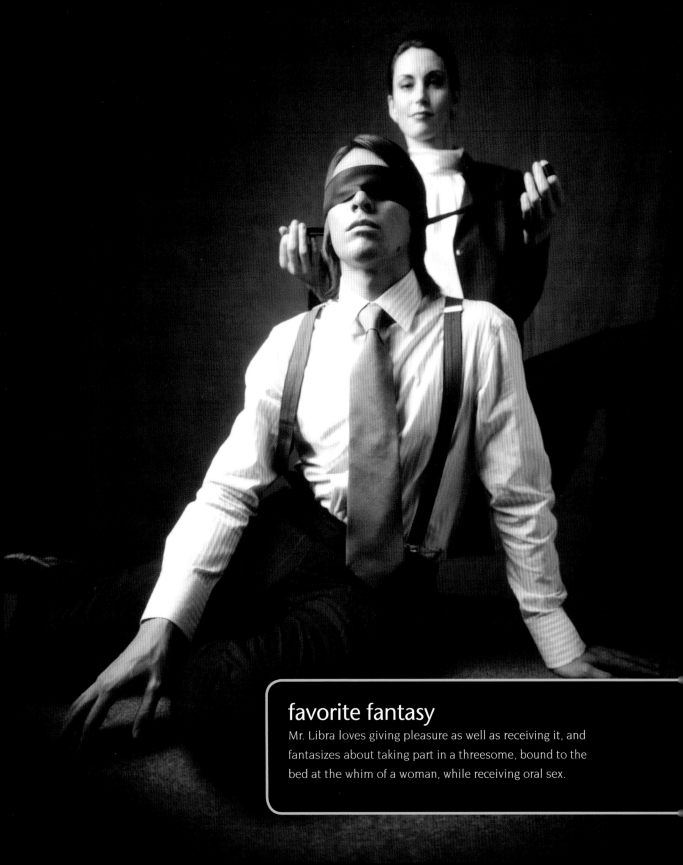

favorite fantasy

Mr. Libra loves giving pleasure as well as receiving it, and fantasizes about taking part in a threesome, bound to the bed at the whim of a woman, while receiving oral sex.

SEDUCTIVE SILK

Utterly romantic dinners for two stimulate his libido while he fingers your naked thighs or silk-stockinged leg and listens to your suggestive words. Mr. Libra has a thing about clothes, and sometimes will even have fun wearing your thong while having sex. Although he's up for a sexy striptease now and then, he's very sensitive about naked bodies, and the faintest flaw or hint of imperfection will instantly turn him off. He's aroused by the feel of silk bras and panties against his penis. He loves to glimpse your breasts, nipples, or buttocks in soft light, but nothing brash or overtly porn. You're the princess of his dreams: innocent, vampish, wicked, and virginal all at once.

TELL ALL

Stare into his eyes and tell him exactly what you're going to do to him. Then do it! Undress him slowly—make it an art—kissing his body as you peel his shirt away from his torso. Keep your clothes on until he's totally naked: by then he'll be so horny he won't even notice you forgot to shave your legs.

Always be utterly feminine, but subtly dominate him and tell him what you want to do next. Quite honestly, he's happy keeping you happy. Put your tongue in his ear, kiss him all over, but don't touch his penis until last. His nipples are super-sensitive, so suck them gently while he masturbates himself. Rub your clitoris all over his buttocks, then turn him over and dominate by sitting astride him. Thrill him by having intercourse while you're still wearing your G-string. Just pull it to one side and he'll adore the feel of the fabric rubbing

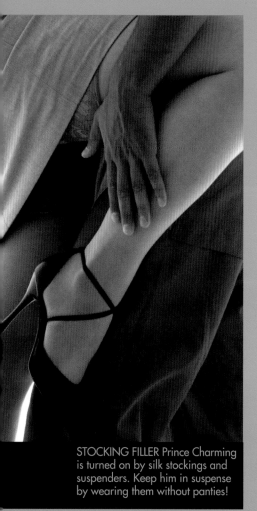

STOCKING FILLER Prince Charming is turned on by silk stockings and suspenders. Keep him in suspense by wearing them without panties!

HORSEPLAY

With a desire to be serenely dominated, Mr. Libra prefers a position where he has visual stimulation to feed his erotic mind and doesn't have to thrash about too much, which might mar the beauty of the performance. The Horseplay sequence provides the perfect balance of great visuals and lazy sensuality for him, and as you get to set the rhythm, he'll have the buzz of knowing you're having a good time too.

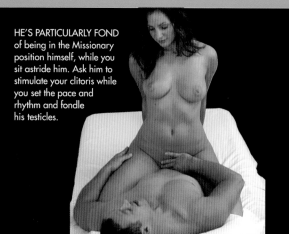

HE'S PARTICULARLY FOND of being in the Missionary position himself, while you sit astride him. Ask him to stimulate your clitoris while you set the pace and rhythm and fondle his testicles.

against his penis. In fact, Mr. Libra is up for anything as long as it gives you pleasure, so start fantasizing now!

PENIS POWER

Mr. Libra's only downside is that he's so insistent that you doesn't really have time to consider whether cunnilingus or anal sex is best for you—that's your decision.

This charmer of the zodiac can be more concerned with getting it up than most other signs. Orgasm can be difficult for

> **Generous** Mr. Libra wants to **please**, but might need a nudge in the right **direction**

please yourself that he doesn't really know how to please you. It's up to you to suggest oral sex, mutual masturbation, *soixante-neuf*, and fetish stuff if that's what turns you on. It's not that he doesn't care, he's just so worried about his image, performance, and romantic vision of perfect union that he him—he's either a long time coming or too fast. The problem is that he lives in his head, an ivory tower where he has to be the perfect Adonis: a difficult ideal to live up to when he knows, deep down, he's just a man like the rest of them. Love his penis but love his mind too; they aren't mutually exclusive.

HIS TOP TURNOFFS

UNSHAVEN ARMPITS

If you've got hairy armpits, get rid of it, or you won't be his "bit of fluff" for long.

BEDROOM TANTRUMS

Mr. Libra wants harmony in bed. He can't bear arguments or weeping women. Get emotional and he'll get out fast.

OUTDATED FASHION

If you're still wearing last year's jeans or dress like a frump, he'd rather fade away into his social crowd than be seen with you.

WALLFLOWER OR BIG-MOUTH

If you can't be as popular as he is, he'll leave you talking to the waiter. If you're an extrovert, remember: good manners and politeness turn him on; swearing and verbal wind-ups don't.

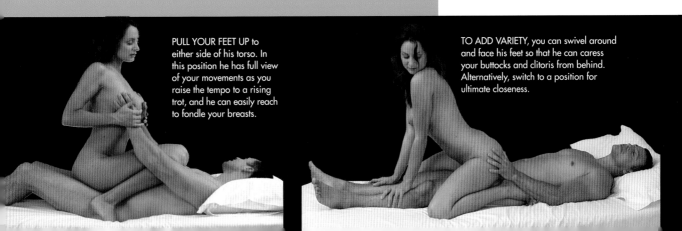

PULL YOUR FEET UP to either side of his torso. In this position he has full view of your movements as you raise the tempo to a rising trot, and he can easily reach to fondle your breasts.

TO ADD VARIETY, you can swivel around and face his feet so that he can caress your buttocks and clitoris from behind. Alternatively, switch to a position for ultimate closeness.

IS THIS THE ONE?

Libra's not an easy catch. Romantic, idealistic, and eternally on the hunt for the perfect partner, no one really lives up to the image. But there are some signs who can play the game and keep the romance going longer than most.

ARIES AND LIBRA

Sexy, challenging, and can last longer than most. Libra adores being dominated, and needs beautiful surroundings and subtle provocation. However, Aries' passion can be exhausting. Always fascinating, and seldom forgettable.

TAURUS AND LIBRA

The bull's down-to-earth nature may disturb Libra's idealistic image of romance. But together you can make a pretty good double act, because you both love the beautiful things in life. Sexually very different, but great for companionship.

GEMINI AND LIBRA

Instant sparks between your sexy and fun-loving minds. Gemini's not emotionally intense and you're both adaptable enough to keep each other guessing. Great for laughter and romance, as long as Libra doesn't always have to compromise.

CANCER AND LIBRA

An unusual blend of sexual spice and almost mystical attraction. Libra's fascinated by the crab's sensitivity and unpredictable responses. Excellent sexual rapport, but Libra will soon tire of Cancer's moodiness.

LEO AND LIBRA

Both enjoy pleasure for the sake of it, as long as it's mingled with glamour and social fun. Libra adores the beautiful things in life; Leo adores the best things in life and living the part. Steamy sexual togetherness, usually long-lasting and sparkling.

VIRGO AND LIBRA

Libra believes Virgo is perfect, and vice versa. But you'll soon accuse each other of all kinds of flaws and will not see eye to eye over work issues. Sexually sizzling, but not an easy relationship for long-term love.

You'll feel an instant rapport, simply because you are so similar. You both love indulging in sexy fantasies and you'll inspire each other's romantic dreams. Harmonious affinity, as long as one of you makes some tangible decisions.

LIBRA AND LIBRA

You bewitch each other with your very differences. Intense and passionate, Libra eventually needs more space and a decent social life. Scorpio would rather draw the curtains and stay at home. Sexually compelling, fantastic for a fling.

SCORPIO AND LIBRA

Utterly romantic duo when you first get together. Both believe you've met the perfect match. But Libra says "we" at every possible moment, while Sagittarius would rather be saying "I." Fun, sex, and magic, if Libra doesn't mind the odd fiery tantrum.

SAGITTARIUS AND LIBRA

The goat has a very different approach to sex and life to Libra. Capricorn thrives on straightforward, no-nonsense sex. Libra wants 24/7 romance. Great for a fling, but there could be power struggles about money, property, and sex.

CAPRICORN AND LIBRA

Fantastic physical rapport, based on erotic mind games. But Aquarius's independence conflicts with Libra's need for a companion. An easy-going relationship, but not so simple once committed. Aquarius says, "I shall," Libra says, "we shouldn't."

AQUARIUS AND LIBRA

Escape into a land of romantic fantasy, dreams, and sex. The fish is looking for the ultimate experience and Libra for the perfect one. But imagination may not be enough to keep you together when the practicalities of life kick in.

PISCES AND LIBRA

AND THE WINNER IS...

If anyone can live up to the day-to-day reality of being the perfect lover of Libra's dreams, then it's probably another Libran. But ironically, it's the elusive, never-quite-sure-what-they're-going-to-do-

next, game-playing partners that will keep Libra happy in the long run. For good, fun-loving mental and sexual rapport, Gemini and Leo are strong contenders, but if someone has to be a winner, then it's Sagittarians who lead the pack, simply for keeping Librans on their romantic toes.

LONG-TERM LOVE WITH LIBRA

The idealists of the zodiac are rarely truly satisfied in love relationships. For a start, they can't help wondering if someone more perfect is going to appear around the next corner. But if you are rational, romantic, and a bit of an independent soul in your own right, then you can be assured of one of the most harmonious and peace-loving partners around.

Librans believe in equality, but on their terms. All must be fair in love and war, but if you can't see that the point they're trying to make is the right one, then they tend to become as self-opinionated as an Aries. Librans desperately want a long-term partner, and if you're prepared to support them in their beliefs, flatter them on a daily basis, and let them waffle about their airy-fairy ideals, you'll have a kind, romantic, and willing partner.

side of life doesn't exist, so don't rub your Libran's face in it. If you want never-ending romance and "togetherness," and can give the scales the approval he or she constantly seek, then he or she is the ultimate partner for you.

GREAT DESIGNS

Libra loves people and beauty, so be prepared to socialize extensively and visit art galleries, and you'll soon be drawing up a perfectly designed plan of your

> If you can **live up to** Libra's high romantic **expectations,** this **perfectionist** may come to believe that you're **the one**

WARTS AND ALL

Relationship is everything to Libra. But for all their romantic idealism, they do have very high standards of etiquette and intellect. The trick is to always give Libra the impression that you are the romantic, perfect creature of their dreams and never let them focus on mundane trivialities and little imperfections (that scar on your toe). Libra would prefer to pretend that

new loft apartment. Librans want to know that you'll be there for them for life if necessary, so say "us" all the time rather than "me" and they will eventually start discussing rings and weddings. Intelligent and civilized, with a laid-back approach to life, Libra is the perfect catch. Do your best to live up to the high expectations and match them for harmonious loving, and you will have a soul mate for life.

LAST STRAW

It's actually easy to turn that romantic light off as quickly as you turned it on with Libra. If you want a Libran to dump you, then there's a simple strategy for getting him or her to do so. Stop trying to live up to the ideal. Let imperfection show—whether it's slobbish behavior, excessive emotion, or criticism of your Libran's lifestyle. Not only can they not bear the idea of being in a relationship with a less-than-perfect partner, but also Librans won't tolerate any suggestion that they might be less than ideal themselves. Wind it all up with a flaming argument, and the balance will well and truly have tipped—out of your favor.

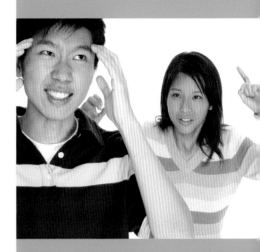

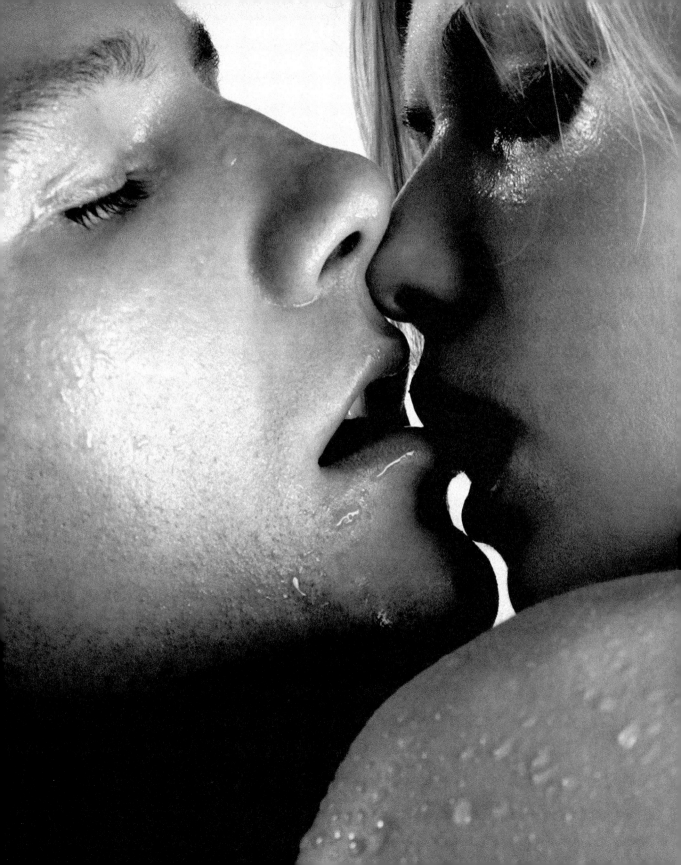

SCORPIO

OCTOBER 24 – NOVEMBER 22

STAR STATS

Ruling planet PLUTO

Signature symbol THE SCORPION

Metal ZIRCON

Stone MALACHITE

Color DEEPEST MAGENTA

Where to find Scorpio Working in the medical profession or on soft porn mags; diving in and out of erotica and naughty lingerie shops.

Hot date Go to see an opera or a Shakespearean tragedy. Scorpio adores passionate life-or-death scenarios.

Needs and desires Scorpio thrives on the taboo side of life, and needs sexual intensity and to totally "burn" with desire for his or her lover.

Top turn-on Mutual masturbation while watching an erotic video.

Sex positions ♀ The Snake

♂ Bestial is Best

Sex toy Stiletto black leather boots.

Sex statistic 86 percent of Scorpios feel lonely during sexual intercourse.

WHAT TO EXPECT WITH SCORPIO

Renowned for being the most erotic, passionate, and lustful sign of the zodiac, the powerful sexual charisma of Scorpio leads them into compelling and sometimes bittersweet love affairs. Smoldering and mysterious, it's all or nothing for this sexually and emotionally intense water sign.

Scorpios are ruled by the god of the underworld, Pluto. And this basically sums them up! The dark side of love and life is far more fascinating to Scorpio than the light. The taboo is so much more enticing than the accepted. They see intimate passion and the complexity of brooding feelings and emotions as theatrical experiences that aren't to be missed. Scorpions are shrewd and instinctively aware of the sexual intensity beneath the veneer of romance and love relationships.

JEALOUSY

If they want you to fall under their spell, they'll suffer hellfire and dangerous liaisons to get you. But there is a downside: this fixed water sign is stubborn, intuitive, and possessive. What they own is for keeps, and their jealousy and manipulative games are renowned. Because they need to feel in control of the sexual stakes, they're the most erotic, compelling, and wicked sign of the zodiac. Once you've been in a relationship with a Scorpio, it's hard to get the sign out of your mind.

BORN EROTIC

Scorpios aren't true sensualists like Taureans. They're seeking an out-of-this-world encounter rather than simple orgasmic pleasure. They have a secret longing for complete and utter merging of bodies, to reconnect with their spiritual selves or surrender to the cosmos. That's why they invest not only their bodies but also their hearts and souls in every sexual relationship. In fact, Scorpios are born erotic. They are beguiling, dark, and unfathomable. Demanding and sexually insatiable, when they are truly in love, they'll move mountains to be at your side.

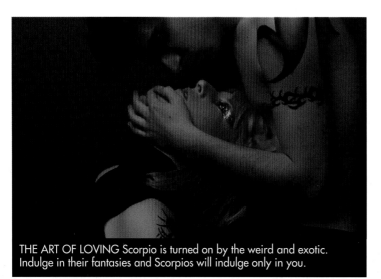

THE ART OF LOVING Scorpio is turned on by the weird and exotic. Indulge in their fantasies and Scorpios will indulge only in you.

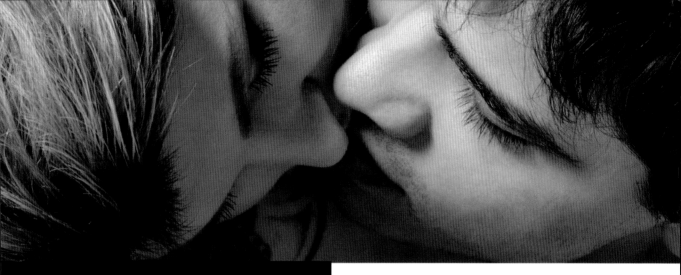

THE SCORPIO MAN

Mysterious and hypnotic, his steely gaze is as sexy as his smile. Notoriously smoldering with passion, he's neither blatant nor macho, and he prefers to seduce you in silence. He's got big opinions about sex, love, money, and power and what will turn you on. He always knows, somehow. However, private parts really are private to this man, and so are your lovemaking antics. Mr. Scorpio is as steamy, volatile, and potent as any fiery lover, but his energy is controlled and contained. He takes his time, likes to dominate, tangles the sheets, and involves his feelings. He's looking for a compelling sexual experience, even though his predatory sexual antics when young give him a bad name. In fact, his penis power is as famous as the Scorpio sting in his tail. But it's all full-blown passion, so make sure that you're as serious about his body and his emotions as he is.

THE SCORPIO WOMAN

The zodiac's *femme fatale* seeks an all-consuming sexual experience, laced with money and power. So if you've got a loaded wallet, make sure you have a loaded sex drive to mat~ She needs to

Volati ̄ ̄io
offers
or-n

feel in control of the love gar ̄ ̄ in and out of bed. Expect power struggles and erotic bliss from this willful, enigmatic woman. She wants to possess and be possessed—she owns you, you own her, and she's looking for a deep erotic connection. Torrid affairs don't scare her, nor does taboo sex.

SCORPIO IN A NUTSHELL

KEYWORDS Erotic; passionate; extremist; stubborn; mysterious; manipulative; jealous; intense; compulsive

LIKES X-rated sex and everything erotic; money; power; intimacy; probing people's minds

DISLIKES Superficiality; niceties; gossiping; being told what to do

TRACKING DOWN YOUR SCORPIO

The smooth-operator of the zodiac isn't easy to find. After all, Scorpio is skilled in the art of cloak and dagger. If you come on to them first, they'll retreat at once. Tracking them down in the corridors of power is possible, or is that enigmatic loner at the bar a Scorpio? Don't ask; wait to be seduced and see.

Scorpios are attracted to money, like their opposite sign, Taurus, but for a slightly different reason: the bull gets off on a feeling of security with money around, but the scorpion gets off on a sense of the power it gives them to do what they want. A need to feel invincible is what drives Scorpios into professions where they can be at the top. You'll often find them working behind the scenes, organizing and controlling teams of people. But they prefer to build their own private empire.

The Scorpio cool head, magnetic aura, and guarded private life gives them the space to work diligently to the top. Single-minded and passionate about everything they do, Scorpios will ruthlessly give up an ordinary lifestyle in their quest for power. They often have informers to keep them posted about what's going on behind the scenes and who is doing what to whom.

> Be prepared to take a **walk on the dark side** of life if you're after this **mysterious** sign

STING IN THE TAIL

Their famous sting in the tail is put to use more often in the workplace than anywhere else.

INTRIGUE

Scorpios often involve themselves in the world of crime or unusual research into taboo subjects like pornography and religious or secret cults. This deeply secretive sign is drawn

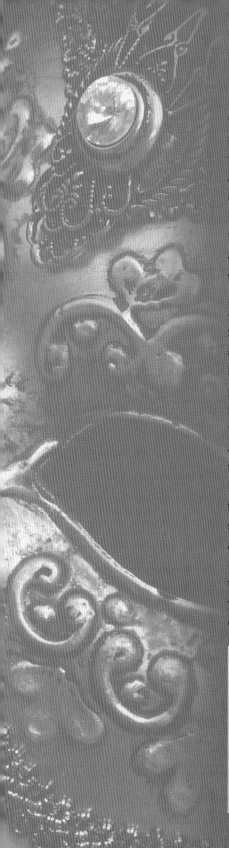

to industrial espionage, where they can use their probing minds to uncover the truth. Both sexes are up for intrigue, and often go on "murder-mystery" or "ghost-hunting" weekends. They find the occult, esoteric subjects and anything to do with sex, money, death, and drama fascinating.

SILENT BROODING TYPE

Socially, Scorpio isn't the most gregarious of signs. Traditionally known for being rather sexually predatory and a bit of a control freak, you can spot Scorpios by their suspicious, brooding attitude to everyone around them. However, attempting to liven them up is the last thing to do. Play the same game, smolder with mystery, and act cool and hard to fathom as if you've more hidden power than a nuclear reactor, and you'll soon draw their probing curiosity in your direction.

PLACES TO LOOK

SEX SHOPS

Their fascination for the taboo and their sexual eccentricity draws them into those purple-colored emporiums. Make sure you're seen investigating the most obscene dildo yet.

DARK BARS AND NIGHTCLUBS

Scorpio is attracted to the dark. Their nocturnal habits involve sophisticated haunts, cool music bars, and private clubs.

THEATER OR OPERA

Hang out at your local theater or become an opera buff. Scorpios are drawn to black comedies, harrowing tales of sorrow, and macabre deeds of darkness.

CORRIDORS OF POWER

Hard to spot. But look like you mean business, and they'll be looking out for you.

SCORPIO TOP TEN CAREERS

1	Headhunter	6	Tax collector/Tax consultant
2	Industrial spy	7	Researcher
3	Film censor	8	Psychotherapist
4	Criminologist	9	Pathologist
5	Insurance investigator	10	Archaeologist

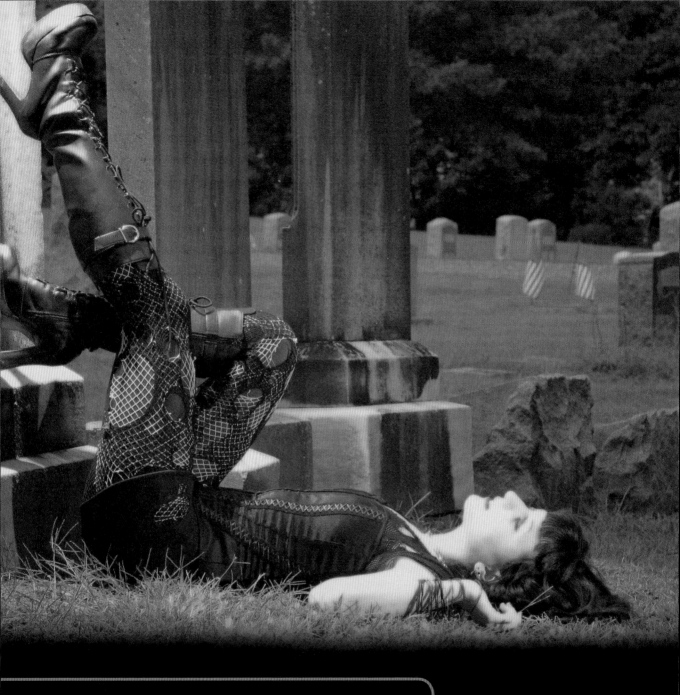

favorite fantasy

Miss Scorpio thrills to the lure of dark places and forbidden
things and loves the idea of unleashing her wicked side with
S&M bondage in a churchyard followed by sex on a grave.

WHAT WORKS FOR HER

Half measures of sex aren't enough for the diva of passion and drama: she needs lashings of attention and total involvement. Her mysterious aura will keep you lusting after her, but she'll keep you at arm's length until she's ready to strike. Miss Scorpio oozes a sultry, come-on quality that is simply compelling.

Miss Scorpio's mistrust of all things includes you. Until she's probed and sussed you out in her own dark way, she's not going to fall into that bed. However sexually aware she is, the Scorpio woman needs to know someone thoroughly before she gives too much away about herself. And that includes intimacy and her sexual secrets. Emotional intensity, drama, and love go hand in hand for her, but she will only express these emotions with someone who can understand her passion for transformative relationships.

> Miss Scorpio will penetrate **your mind** long before you can even think about **penetrating** her

HYPNOTIC

Her sexual expression is smoldering and hypnotic. Powerful and extreme, she's most turned on when you submit to her ways. Conveying an aura of powerful and erotic intensity, she's envied by many women and desired by many men. With a profound insight into her sexual needs, she's one of the most lustful and enriching of lovers. Miss Scorpio's arousal is forceful, intense, and serious, and a physical and emotional theatrical performance is absolutely essential to her orgasmic energy flow.

HOW TO MAKE HER HORNY

Once you know you're welcome in Scorpio's acutely private sexual world, you won't really need much sex-manual advice! Indeed, more than any other sign of the zodiac, she's likely to want to be in control of the foreplay. The secret is to let her take the lead; the more she dominates, the hornier she gets. Scorpio's astro erogenous zone begins at the cleft of her buttocks leading up and around to her vulva. In fact, she's wired for permanent sexual arousal. To really boost her high sex drive, lick, tongue, or nibble her buttocks, then brush your fingers down and around her anus toward her clitoris and back again and she'll be in raptures. She'll also find it a big turn-on if you follow this up by tracing the same path with the tip of your penis, and then let her lead the way.

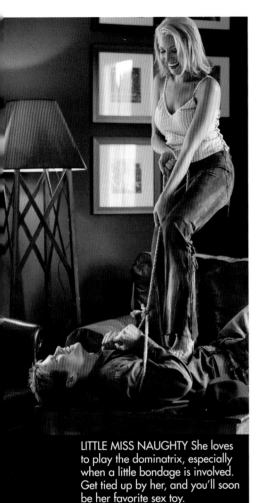

LITTLE MISS NAUGHTY She loves to play the dominatrix, especially when a little bondage is involved. Get tied up by her, and you'll soon be her favorite sex toy.

DARK SOPHISTICATION

The *femme fatale* of the zodiac is turned on by enigmatic or mysterious encounters, secret liaisons, other women's lovers, secret affairs, and seduction for the sake of it. Kissing in the dark or masturbating each other in the back row of the cinema is the kind of after-hours action that your Scorpio woman craves. Men who'd literally die for her make her feel "sin-sational," and serious money, seriously rich rogues, and smooth-operators are sexual turn-ons too. Erotic underwear, erotic books and films, and the dark side of life give her a buzz. But her greatest sexual trigger is a sense of power, so never forget that she prefers to play the dominant role.

Miss Scorpio enjoys the kick of being the "Madame" in charge of sophisticated gentle bondage. Let her tie you naked to a chair with silk scarves or stockings. Ask her to smother your penis with her favorite champagne or honey and then let her lick or suck it all off, slowly. Next, suggest she sit astride you and rub her clitoris against your belly and penis, without penetration. Finding wicked or dangerous locations is also one of her favorite erotic triggers. Let her masturbate you in the kitchen at a friend's house while everyone's eating dinner, or visit a deserted churchyard at night and have oral sex under the moonlight.

EMOTIONAL SEX DRIVE

Scorpio's issue with power is because she feels so vulnerable. And she reacts emotionally and excessively to every word, move, action, and orgasm you have. Her possessive temperament means she's unlikely to get involved in threesomes or group sex. She

THE SNAKE

You lie on your back on the bed or floor. She kneels astride your upper belly, facing your feet—the naughtiness of rear-entry sex is a big turn-on. Moisten the cleft of her buttocks with your fingers or place your hands up and through her legs to stimulate her clitoris. This position allows her to move her buttocks back over your face when she feels ready for oral sex, *soixante-neuf* style, with her on top.

ASK HER TO SQUAT DOWN GENTLY onto your penis, still facing in the direction of your feet. She doesn't need to see your face to know you'll be in sexual heaven!

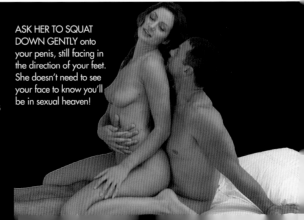

HER TOP TURNOFFS

BEING SUBMISSIVE
If she's not on top or in control of the rhythm, then she won't find it easy to orgasm.

INDECISIVENESS
She expects her lover to be as sure of himself as he is of her. Never "hum and hah" about dates or about having spontaneous sex—just get on with it.

PENNILESS ARTISTS
If you don't have a lot of money, never admit it. This lady believes that money, sex, and power go together. If you're a starving artist, you'd better get famous quick.

LIGHTWEIGHTS
Scorpio is serious about love and life. She likes a laugh, but she doesn't want superficiality or wisecracks in the sack.

can lunge from jealous mistrust to complete and utter abandon. Her polarities are so perverse that she can be both obsessively erotic and totally cold. She needs to learn that power turns her on, and what she's seeking in sexual intimacy is power for herself, not control over her partner.

DRAMA QUEEN
However, Miss Scorpio knows that she also has the power to get away with virtually anything she chooses. It's not that she's ruthless, but she's a bit of a drama queen about her sexual needs. Scorpios have been known to steal other women's lovers and have double standards. She may insist on complete fidelity from you when she's capable of sexual betrayal herself. She's also fond of storming off saying she'll never see you again, just to see if she can win you back

with her erotic, sultry seduction. She usually does. In fact, Scorpio sometimes withholds sex as an emotional weapon or offers it as bribe in her battle for survival and power in any relationship.

DARK PLEASURES
Her curiosity about the dark side of life may encourage her to try any perverse or obscure sexual position or fetish. She usually experiments with anal sex at some point in her life, although she's likely to prefer taking on a dominatrix role and playing out her S&M fantasies: walking over your back and bottom in spiky heels, spanking you, or using a dildo to give you anal sex. She'll enjoy masturbating in front of you; wearing rubber, leather, or fur; and dressing you up in erotic lingerie or fetish clothes. Her imagination knows no bounds, nor does her sexual extremism.

LET HER SET THE PACE and depth of penetration while she caresses your testicles. She likes clitoral stimulation at the same time as hard penetration, and often prefers to masturbate herself to orgasm.

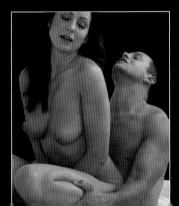

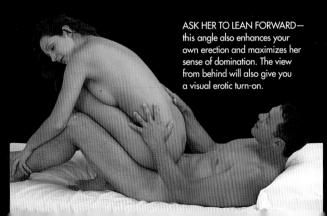

ASK HER TO LEAN FORWARD— this angle also enhances your own erection and maximizes her sense of domination. The view from behind will also give you a visual erotic turn-on.

WHAT WORKS FOR HIM

For all his potent sex drive, this man is looking for a deeply transformative sexual experiences. Sex is not just about pleasure or showing off his penis (although he can go on a Casanova trip when young); it's a deeper erotic and symbolic connection to his own power. Sex is not a goal in itself; power is.

> Secretly **vulnerable**, he needs to find a woman who can **point him in the direction** of his **soul** as well as his **penis**

Most of all, Scorpio needs to feel in control and to sexually dominate you to be aroused. The more mysterious you are, the more he'll want to have you. And the more likely you are both to be caught in the act, the better his orgasm. On first dates, make sure that you know a lot about money, sex, and power issues, and that you can discuss the masturbatory habits of monks without flinching. Mr. Scorpio loves dangerously. His libido is all about tangled sheets, dark alleyways, secret meetings, sexual vamps, and smoldering all-night sex marathons.

MYSTERY MAN

When he appears all aloof and mysterious, he's actually figuring you out. Don't let him know all your sex secrets or fantasies too soon—he likes to probe, and the more enigmatic you are, the more he'll hang around. He is possessive though, and incredibly jealous. He might not show it, but if you flirt or don't look as if you're having the best sex ever with him, he'll drop you instantly.

HOW TO MAKE HIM HORNY

Not that difficult. If he's got the hots for you, then he's already horny. But to help him on the way, he thrives on a sensual and erotic buttock massage: this area is Mr. Scorpio's prime astro-erogenous zone. Start off using the palm of your hands with firm, flat strokes, interspersed with lighter, teasing brushes over the sensitive skin. Then add in your fingers to vary the sensations, then your lips, and finally your tongue. Use swirling patterns and unpredictable movements to heighten the erotic sensations. Make sure that you pay some teasing attention to the cleft of his anus too. At the same time, slowly push your hand down beneath his belly and stroke his penis—he likes it if you get straight to the point! By then, he'll probably prefer to take total control of the proceedings, and dominate you

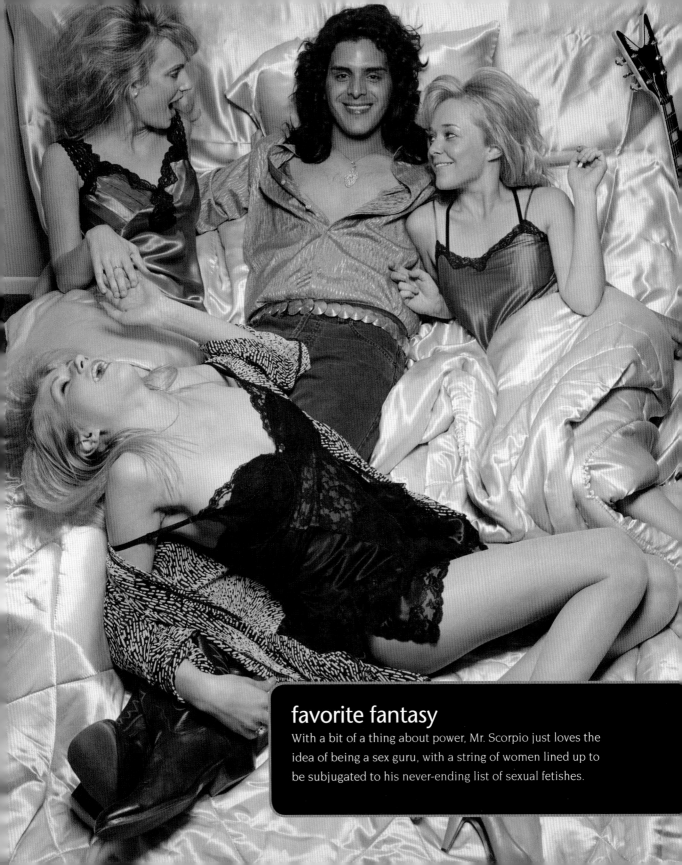

favorite fantasy

With a bit of a thing about power, Mr. Scorpio just loves the
idea of being a sex guru, with a string of women lined up to
be subjugated to his never-ending list of sexual fetishes.

DEMANDING LOVER

Scorpio's desire for sex is pretty much a 24/7 event. In fact, if he's not doing it every day, he's thinking about it. He's proud of his morning-till-night erections and is quite capable of having sex with any available woman who takes his fancy. But when he does fall in love, he falls hard. This man wields power and needs to feel empowered through his sexual performance.

SEXUAL EXTREMIST

You must be prepared to try out everything from sex in taboo places to S&M and masturbation competitions. Scorpio is born with a sexual mind. And if you can match him for spontaneity, variety, and wickedness, he'll be forever at your side. However, once Scorpio has lured you into his net, it's very hard to get out again. Possessive and jealous, he gets perversely turned on by seeing you flirt with other men, and it's this perverted side that causes him the most trouble. Suspicious to the extreme, he'll check your cell phone for coded numbers and expect you to drop everything for a quick bonk in his lunch-hour. Beware though, Scorpio can be one of the most unfaithful men in the zodiac, simply because he's on a quest to prove something to himself.

CONTROL FREAK

Mr. Scorpio likes to take control of the sexual action. But keep one step ahead of him and he'll secretly love your inventiveness. Visit him at work when everyone's

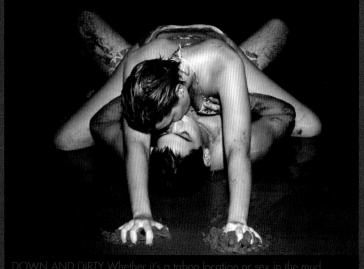

DOWN AND DIRTY Whether it's a taboo location or sex in the mud, outrageous Mr. Scorpio wants to play the filthiest games of all.

BESTIAL IS BEST

With his desire to dominate, your Scorpio prefers rear-entry, doggy-style sex. This position allows for maximum penetration, is a visual stimulus for Mr. Scorpio, and also enables you to take control of your own orgasm. Your sexily submissive posture is guaranteed to send his libido into overdrive. You can move from this sequence into other more complex domination positions.

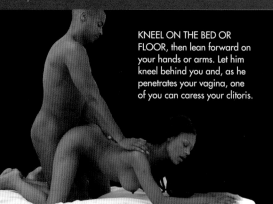

KNEEL ON THE BED OR FLOOR, then lean forward on your hands or arms. Let him kneel behind you and, as he penetrates your vagina, one of you can caress your clitoris.

left, and have sex on the office desk. Show him erotic photos, especially of women making love, while you masturbate him. Take him on a mystery tour—visit some wild and windy spot in the country and have sex in the rain. Give him oral sex while

He's **happy** to spend time with you **watching porn**, reading erotica, and acting out **fantasies**

he's talking on the phone, or play the vamp and have doggy-style sex on the floor with you wearing long black gloves. Don't orgasm until he does: the more restrained and apparently shy you are during foreplay, the more sex he'll want. Wear a G-string and let him trace the string with his lips and tongue.

MASTURBATION

Mr. Scorpio is fond of lots of foreplay and long hard penetration. He's also up for anal sex if you are, and will try anything once. He needs variety, drama, and theatrical sex. But not an audience—although he will try out threesomes if you're happy for another woman to be in on the equation. One of his greatest turn-ons is mutual masturbation. And he's likely to spend a lot of time doing it alone. Scorpio's dark side lies in his fascination with S&M and his macabre fantasies ranging from bestiality to vampirism.

HIS TOP TURN OFFS

COCK-TEASERS
Talking about sex rather than doing it is a no-no. If you're a bit of a cock-tease, stay away from this permanently cocked man.

SUGAR AND NICENESS
Squeaky clean, good girls just don't turn him on and that's that. You have to know what filth is and get dirty with it.

ROMANTIC TWADDLE
I'm afraid so. He knows it's all an illusion, and he's just a man with a penis and that's the end of the story.

WEAKNESS
Compassionate he is, but he won't put up with feeble or lazy people. If you get yourself into a mess, you'd better sort it out—he won't hang around.

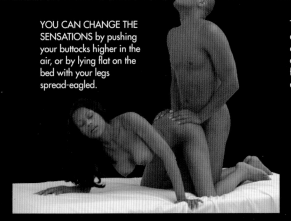

YOU CAN CHANGE THE SENSATIONS by pushing your buttocks higher in the air, or by lying flat on the bed with your legs spread-eagled.

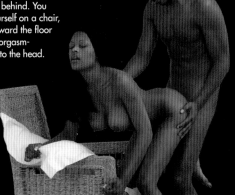

TRY STANDING UPRIGHT as he enters you from behind. You can support yourself on a chair, or bend over toward the floor for the ultimate orgasm-enhancing rush to the head.

IS THIS THE ONE?

Scorpio's looking for a match in sexual intensity and a powerful purpose in life. It's all-or-nothing, serious stuff when it comes to long-term relationships, but for a brief affair, well, virtually anyone goes in Scorpio's wicked book.

ARIES AND SCORPIO

Scorpio can be too intense and emotional for the ram's more dynamic and extrovert style. You will have an exhilarating sex life, but Scorpio's dark outlook on life doesn't mix well with Aries' light one.

TAURUS AND SCORPIO

Natural opposites of the zodiac always attract. The sexual tension between you will be like a magnet—a love-hate relationship in the extreme. Erotic fascination for each other, but possessive and emotionally challenging.

GEMINI AND SCORPIO

Scorpio's intrigued by Gemini's ambiguous personality, and Gemini is fascinated by Scorpio's secret side. However, Gemini will feel stifled by all that intense closeness, and Scorpio will think Gemini too shallow. Not easy in the long-term.

CANCER AND SCORPIO

Fascinated by one another's very private nature, you'll crave complete emotional closeness and be sexually dedicated to each other. Good long-term relationship potential, but may not be as challenging as Scorpio desires.

LEO AND SCORPIO

Leo's flirtatious; Scorpio's intensely serious and difficult to satisfy. Yet there's a very powerful attraction between you that won't go away. A highly compelling sexual union and a lasting success, if Leo doesn't make Scorpio jealous.

VIRGO AND SCORPIO

Virgo's searching for an ordered love life. Scorpio prefers a more chaotic and cathartic approach to relationships. Scorpio will eventually feel unfulfilled by Virgo's cool approach to sex. Good for a sexy fling; more difficult for long-term love.

Libra wants the **perfect relationship**, and loves being subjected to Scorpio's **intense** mystical and sexual power. But a very different lifestyle approach. Scorpio wants **all or nothing**, Libra wants to be **free**, in case someone more perfect shows up.

LIBRA AND SCORPIO

An **instant affinity**, but you could end up playing too many **power games**. Exciting and **intense** if you enjoy the element of **danger** of who can outwit or out-pleasure the other. A sexy, **wicked affair**, but watch out for love triangles.

SCORPIO AND SCORPIO

Archers need to feel free to **come and go** when they please. Scorpios **need to know** exactly what the archer's doing and where. **Sexually exciting** and great for a **short-term fling**, but runs into problems when the archer **escapes** abroad.

SAGITTARIUS AND SCORPIO

You're both **aroused** by **sexual power**, and there could be conflicts about who's **in control**. Capricorn learns from Scorpio's passion, and Scorpio from the goat's **pragmatism**. A **passionate commitment** together to rule the world.

CAPRICORN AND SCORPIO

Often a highly **magnetic** and **erotic** relationship. But Scorpio wants **total involvement** and Aquarius isn't interested in exclusivity. Great for an **unconventional** and sexy affair, if Scorpios can dump their **jealous streak**. Difficult long-term.

AQUARIUS AND SCORPIO

Sexually perfect. But the fish is a social animal and likes to **gossip** about your bedroom antics, while Scorpio's **discreet** and won't want your intimate life **broadcast** around town. Good for **emotional affinity**, but lifestyle needs are very different.

PISCES AND SCORPIO

AND THE WINNER IS...

Aquarius, Gemini, and Libra, are ultimately too

LONG-TERM LOVE WITH SCORPIO

If you think you can handle this emotional, powerful, and erotic sign, take care. Long-term, Scorpios aren't easy partners. They desperately want commitment, but to Scorpios, commitment doesn't mean fidelity. For them, anyway: there's always the erotic lure of temptation. Yet, with tolerance and understanding, this could be one of the most creative and erotic relationships ever.

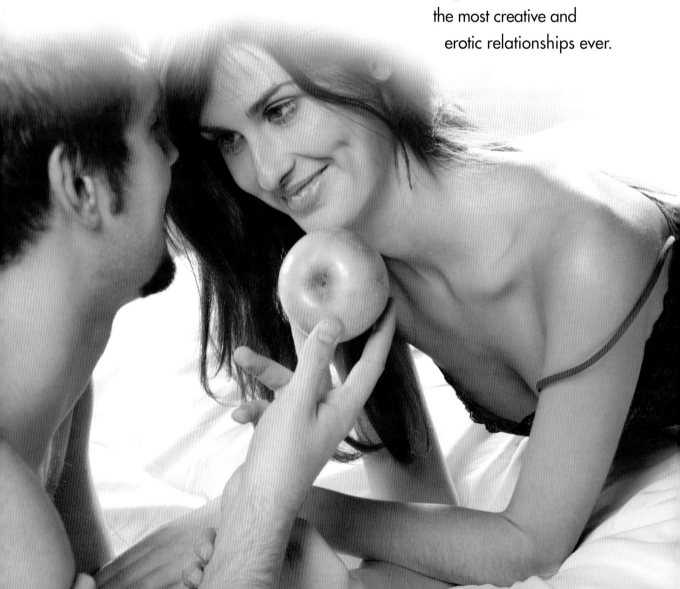

For all Scorpios' double standards, once they commit themselves to you then you can be assured of a transformative, long-term, creative relationship. But you must be emotionally honest and have a serious interest in making something of your life too. Although you might be the love of their lives, they will need to keep a side of themselves private, so respect their time alone by giving them lots of space and doing your

can be trusted, then Scorpios will put their hearts into making that trust work both ways. That's a greater reward than anything else, because it means they're with you for life. Believe in their insights, side with them when the world gets tough, never wound their vulnerable pride, and you can look forward to building a successful empire together. They can't be tamed or caged, but Scorpios do respond to exclusive love and understanding.

> # Commitment with Scorpio means just that: a total merging of minds, bodies, and souls

own thing too. However, be ready to jump to attention when Scorpio's feeling emotionally in need of intimacy. Never forget that this star-sign lives and breathes through an intense sexual relationship.

GREEN EYES

Scorpio's notorious jealousy is a reaction to a fear of rejection. And they won't tolerate betrayal from a partner. However, if you can really and truly show you

DARK AND LIGHT

Show that you are willing to transform your life at the drop of a hat, be creative and experimental in your sex life, and Scorpios will realize that they have at last met their match. To keep scorpions from straying, you must be as obsessed with them as they are with you. They need a partner who has a wry sense of humor too, who can laugh at the dark side of life as much as the light.

THE STING

It's not that hard to get Scorpio to dump you: if they have any reason to suspect you of betrayal, they won't stand for it. So use their double standards against them—make them doubt your fidelity and they'll be gone. Scorpios link inconsistency with unfaithfulness, so be late from work, flirt with all their friends, don't answer their phone calls, and let them catch you texting someone else and refuse to show them the screen. And the *pièce de résistance?* Accuse them of having an affair themselves. You're using their secret vulnerability against them: as soon as they think you don't trust them, how could they possibly trust you? Result: one crushed scorpion.

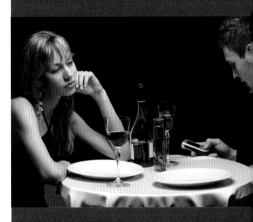

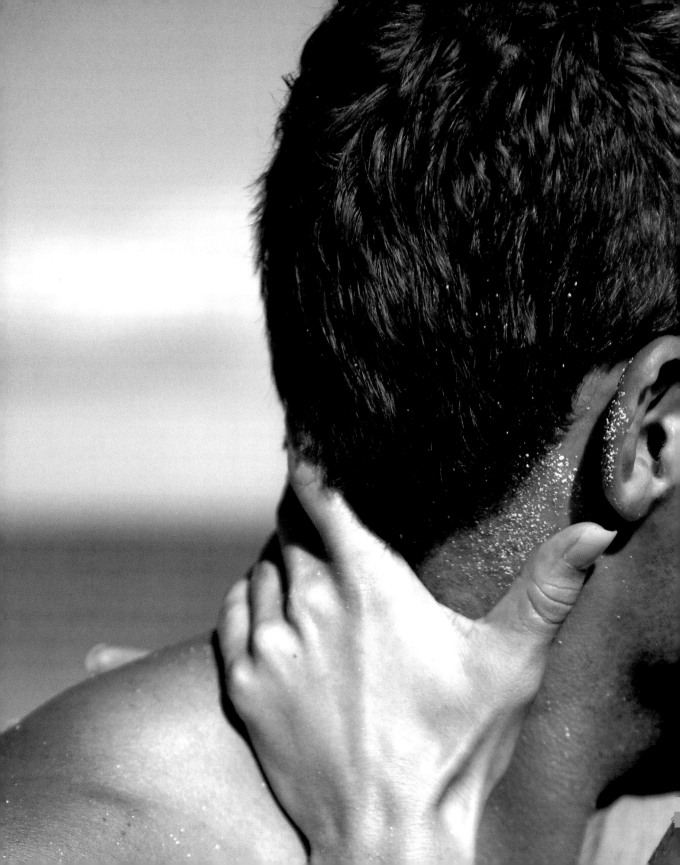

SAGITTARIUS

NOVEMBER 23 – DECEMBER 21

STAR STATS

Ruling planet JUPITER
Signature symbol THE ARCHER
Metal TIN
Stone TURQUOISE
Color MIDNIGHT BLUE

Where to find Sagittarius Comedy shows, horse-riding centers, surfing the breakers, or backpacking around the world.

Hot date Fly to a foreign city and back again on the same day. Archers adore the pace and excitement of travel.

Needs and desires Hilarious and fun-loving, Sagittarius needs plenty of freedom and spontaneous sexual excitement.

Top turn-on Sex in the great outdoors or oral sex in the car.

Sex positions ♀ The Tiger
♂ Swivel Stick

Sex toy Feather.

Sex statistic 90 percent of Sagittarians fantasize about orgies.

WHAT TO EXPECT WITH SAGITTARIUS

Adventure-loving Sagittarius is one of the most extrovert, hilarious, and idealistic of signs. Direct and spontaneous, they fall in love fast but fall out of it equally fast if they start to feel trapped. Their enthusiasm is infectious and their sexy, debonair charisma gets them noticed everywhere they go.

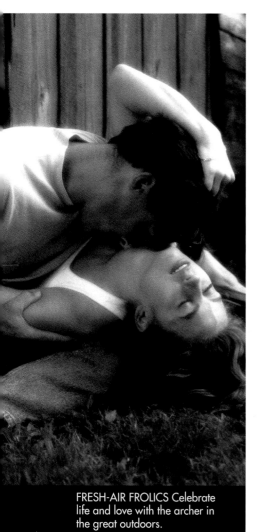

FRESH-AIR FROLICS Celebrate life and love with the archer in the great outdoors.

Sagittarius is ruled by Jupiter, the god of expansion and optimism. This fiery god was also notoriously promiscuous, which is why archers have a bit of a reputation for spreading themselves around. But it's their never-ending quest for romance, excitement, and meaning in both love and life that motivates them to fall for strangers and lead independent lives. Freedom-lovers, they hate to be tied down to anything, whether it's promising to meet you on a date next week (after all they might have changed their minds by then) or a case of committing themselves to a long-term relationship. With boundless energy and a constant desire to keep moving on, you can never be sure where they'll be at any moment of the day. Romantic and rampant, they are totally frank about their sexual needs and believe sex is a celebration of life.

UNCONVENTIONAL

If you're on the lookout for a conventional relationship, then stay away from Sagittarius. They roam, play, and are looking for a freedom-loving traveling companion—well for a while anyway. In fact, the secret of Sagittarians is that they prefer brief encounters and the spirit of adventurous sex to commitment and 2.5 children.

WILD ROVER

Upfront and blunt, the archer is also brilliant at seduction. Sagittarians instinctively know how to make you smile and how to turn you on. However, they do exaggerate the facts and can be the most unreliable sign in the zodiac. But if you're up for fun, crazy romance and totally uninhibited sex, then this is the sign for you. These are wild rovers, but if you're one as well, this could be the most fun and sexy relationship ever.

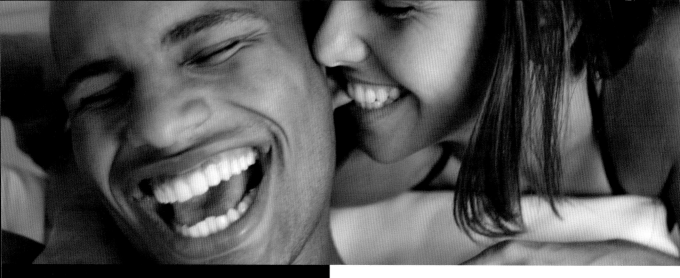

THE SAGITTARIUS MAN

With a fiery belief that he's the best stud around, it's hard not to fall for this funny, adventurous man. The crusader of the zodiac makes a lot of noise. He's popular in his social circle, and usually has

> He considers his **body** to be **magnificent**, and loves to be **naked**

more women friends than he does male. Daring, audacious, and raunchy, he'll laugh about his body, express his sexual needs without embarrassment, and have sex on his mind nearly all day. What about the night? That's play time. He's after fiery, imaginative sex, not serious emotional closeness.

THE SAGITTARIUS WOMAN

This is one impatient lady. Sex has to be now, when she wants it, and if she has to wait too long for it then she'll end up getting bored and moving on to another seductive smile. Miss Archer is impatient for more of everything and insatiably hungry for sexual excitement. Passionate and exotic, she's liable to drag you off for an utterly wild afternoon of adventure and sex in the great outdoors. The more exciting the relationship, the longer it will last. Communication is also very important to her, so talk all night across the pillow (in between lots of oral sex, of course), and she'll still be on the phone or e-mailing sexy messages to you all through the day. And whether you are single, attached to someone else, or the world's most glamorous eligible celebrity, as long as you've got a rampant sex drive to match hers, this wild-roving lady will be up for fun.

SAGITTARIUS IN A NUTSHELL

KEYWORDS Optimistic; adventurous; impulsive; extravagant; high-spirited; freedom-loving; flashy; versatile

LIKES Traveling; knowing all the best people; being seen in the best places; sex outdoors; having fun

DISLIKES Making promises; possessive lovers; being serious

TRACKING DOWN YOUR SAGITTARIUS

Tracking them down isn't difficult, but it's going to be hard to keep up with them. Always on the move, you're more likely to meet the archer by accident than by design. However, if you love traveling and get out and about as much as they do, you're certain to bump into Sagittarians without even trying.

Sagittarius wants action, and this restless, mutable sign won't enjoy being trapped in a confined space from 9 to 5, unless it's up in the clouds in a Learjet. Sagittarians prefer wheeling and dealing. When they take risks they usually fall on their feet, win new accounts, or clinch a deal, simply because they're astute enough to be in the right place at the right time.

Sagittarians **always want** to be moving on to **new places,** so **act fast** or be left behind

unexpected challenges and adventurous projects to ritual and routine, and they like to be surrounded by people who share their enormous visions or are equally goal oriented. Some people call them lucky, but the archers are quick to learn who and what can lead them to that pot of gold.

GO-GETTERS

Go-getting, dynamic, and quick-witted, Sagittarians make great crusaders or marketeers. They can persuade anyone to do anything when they're on form, and excel at selling or buying,

ON YOUR TRAVELS

Stroll around any airport lounge, take a ride on a horse, or set off on a safari trip and you're bound to come across a Sagittarius. Blessed with spirited energy, the archer enjoys traveling more than anything else. But Sagittarians usually travel light, so if you bump into them in a hotel bar, you can be pretty sure they're only there for one night. They love gambling and taking risks by indulging in dangerous sports like skydiving, mountaineering, jet-skiing, or bareback riding. With an intuitive feeling that luck's on their side, Sagittarians are easily tempted by the lure of roulette wheels and horse racing.

PEOPLE IN HIGH PLACES

Sagittarius adores glamour, success, and people who are larger-than-life. Celebrities fall into this category, and you can be sure they know someone in the news: a Hungarian prince, an Australian outback hero, a Russian poet, or a Chinese mystic. In fact, the more you join in the jet set or mingle with the exotic individualists of this world, the more likely it is that you'll get invited to one of Sagittarius's lavish, madcap parties.

PLACES TO LOOK

FOREIGN RESTAURANTS

If they do have time to stop and eat, they're likely to be the ones who can dextrously handle the chopsticks, attack hot chilli without sweating, and talk knowledgeably about anything from Venezuelan cuisine to pigs' brains. The archer is a bit of a snob and likes to be seen in all the most fashionable places.

ABROAD

Get traveling. Anywhere exotic, different, or fashionable. Big cities and the wild outdoors are equally attractive to the archer.

UNIVERSITIES/COLLEGES

Sagittarians often explore life through the mind rather than becoming backpackers. They can make excellent teachers, lecturers, and, of course, the ubiquitous eternal students.

SAGITTARIUS TOP TEN CAREERS

1 Explorer
2 Travel writer
3 Teacher/Lecturer
4 Sales person
5 Travel agent
6 Eternal student
7 Horse trainer
8 Airline pilot
9 Publisher
10 Philosopher

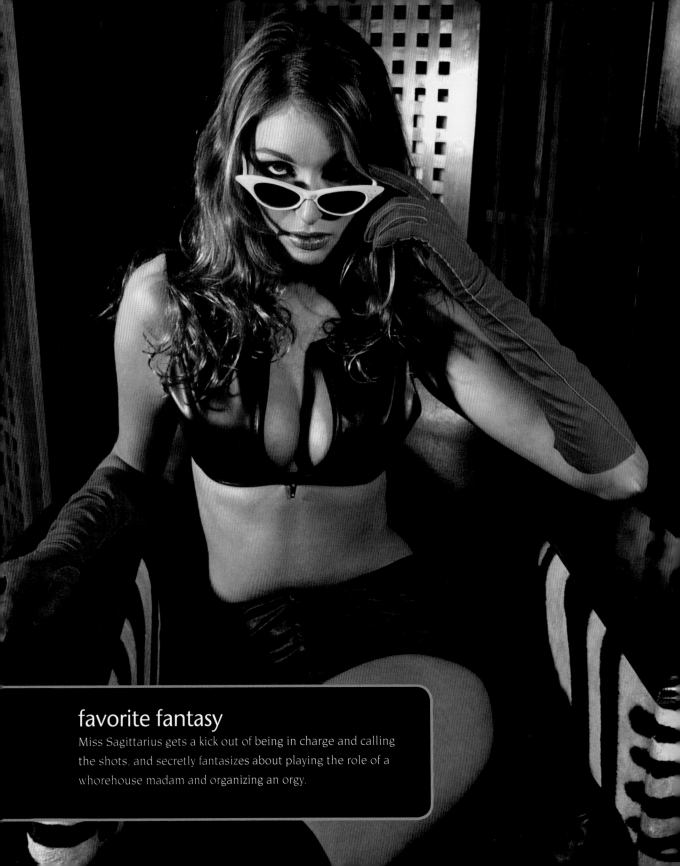

favorite fantasy

Miss Sagittarius gets a kick out of being in charge and calling the shots, and secretly fantasizes about playing the role of a whorehouse madam and organizing an orgy.

WHAT WORKS FOR HER

This independent woman will never be possessed, and really values her sexual freedom. She's a bit like a love virus—totally catchable. Her infectious company, insatiable appetite for romance, and fun-loving attitude make her sizzle with sexiness. Just take care: she'll only be there as long as she wants to be.

An utter romantic, the Sagittarius woman in love is full of optimism and wildly orgasmic. And if she's out of love, she wants to fall right in all over again. Breathtaking and unstoppable, she just wants to celebrate life through sexy fun. Sounds too good to be true? Well, this vitalizing woman does have a tendency to make promises that she can't keep. She's really enthusiastic about going to that party with you; then a few days later, she'll be bored with the idea and make up some excuse about going to Paris on business.

> This **flamboyant** woman is renowned for **flings** with anyone from **rock stars** to freewheelers

SEXUAL FREEDOM

It's drama, glamour, excitement, and the thrill of the chase that are the Sagittarius woman's biggest turn-ons. She'd rather be out there pulling you than waiting for you to chat her up. Romantic fantasy plays a big part in her sexual arousal, and she adores men who are up for wild but brief affairs. She's easily tempted by spontaneous sex with strangers in trains, planes, or among the coats at a party. But if you do get to be more than a one-night stand, feed her desires by having sex in the great outdoors and talking dirty to her whenever you get the chance.

HOW TO MAKE HER HORNY

Uninhibited Sagittarius is turned on by direct, spontaneous foreplay. In fact, she's prepared to come right out with it and tell you exactly what to do—erotic conversations are high on her list of turn-ons. The epicenter of her sexual energy flow is located around her inner thighs, about an inch down from her pubis. Playfully caress, kiss, and lick her there without touching her vulva or clitoris to really drive her wild. Featherlight tracing of your fingers along her inner thighs will send a bolt of pleasure to the right spot! Get into sound effects too. She adores hearing you grunt, moan, talk dirty, and laugh, laugh, laugh. For Miss Sagittarius, sex isn't a matter of serious commitment. It's fun that she's after, and not an emotional meeting of bodies and souls.

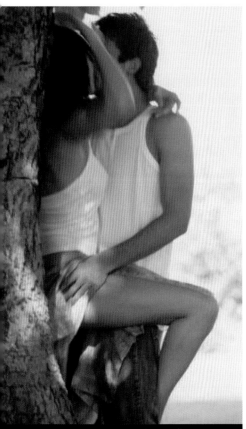

TREE NYMPH Throw all caution to the wind when you're out in the country or the local park and get turned on by the most audacious woman of the zodiac.

EQUALITY

Sagittarius's sexual expression is agile and audacious. Finding a partner to satisfy her extravagant sexuality and wild, demanding sex drive isn't easy. OK, she's up for one-night stands, ships passing in the night, or a brief encounter with a kindred spirit. But she's really looking for a friend and most of all an equal. And sexually she hates to play power games and will flip from submissive to dominant as the mood takes her.

JOYFUL

She wants sex to be a mutually joyful, exciting experience, no strings attached. Throwing herself into uninhibited foreplay, she will abandon herself to her animal instincts and show off her ability for quick orgasms. Oral sex is one of her favorite ways to climax, and she's happy to kneel before you, licking and caressing your penis, the more impulsive and daring the location the better to indulge her desire for spontaneous hot arousal. She fantasizes about voyeurism, so sex in a situation where she might be found out—standing up with her back against a tree as you lick and tongue her clitoris—is a big libido boost.

TALK DIRTY

Keeping Sagittarius happy involves thinking ahead. She's not exactly the type to flop on the sofa watching an erotic video or spend hours gazing into your eyes over a romantic supper. She wants sex whenever she feels like it, and that's that. Sex is dirty—so talk dirty. Tape your voices, sighs, and moans while you're bonking the night away and play it back later while you're in the car. Then have sex

THE TIGER

The Tiger gives her the hard, bestial kind of penetration she likes. Stand in front of a bed, ask her to turn her back and raise herself up on her tiptoes if shorter than you. You stand behind her stroking or kissing her buttocks. Push your penis hard into her vagina, set the pace initially, then let her decide what rhythm is best for her. After this, experimental Miss Sagittarius will want to try every position under the sun.

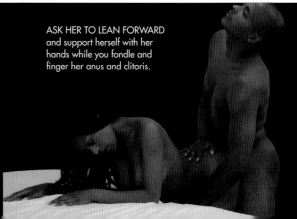

ASK HER TO LEAN FORWARD and support herself with her hands while you fondle and finger her anus and clitoris.

HER TOP TURNOFFS

ROUTINE SEX
She gets bored very quickly with the same techniques or positions—don't ever underestimate her love of experimentation.

LOCKED DOORS
Leave that door open for a quick exit and never tie her down. The more she sees you on a routine basis, the sooner she'll want out.

INTIMACY
She's not concerned with feelings, possessiveness, or the idea of "real intimacy." This fun-loving lady wants to be your "friend" not an extension of you.

SERIOUS MEN
If you take things too personally or don't have a sense of humor, then forget Sagittarius—she'll quickly forget you anyway!

in the lay-by. Unpredictable sex rather than obvious bedtime routines gives her the freedom to flow into sexual oblivion. And she adores space, whether it's a deserted beach, a huge double-king-size bed or a mountaintop. She's quickly turned on if sex is preceded by action or adventure, like horse riding, skinny-dipping, arm-wrestling, or any sporty competition between you. Hard penetrative sex all through the night won't faze her—her energy is stunning—but if you're the type who falls asleep after you orgasm, this lady isn't for you.

ORGIES
The archer is perfectly willing to try out a *ménage à trois*, and will adore taking the lead and showing off her sexual know-how. However, she is a little naive about other people's sexual needs and desires, so

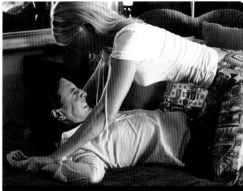

GET SPORTY The energetic archer is up for all kinds of competitive action before sex, like wrestling her partner into submission.

if she insists on anal sex or bondage, make sure the third party is up for that kind of adventure too. True to her explorative urge, if a party turns into an orgy, she'll involve herself totally, moving from a man to a woman to whatever takes her fancy, so that if one partner tires, she can maintain her libido peaks and satisfy her desire for multiple orgasms all night long.

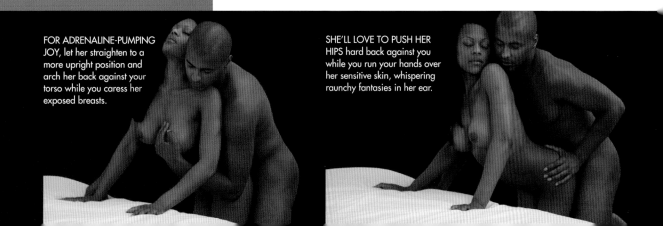

FOR ADRENALINE-PUMPING JOY, let her straighten to a more upright position and arch her back against your torso while you caress her exposed breasts.

SHE'LL LOVE TO PUSH HER HIPS hard back against you while you run your hands over her sensitive skin, whispering raunchy fantasies in her ear.

WHAT WORKS FOR HIM

Mr. Sagittarius comes across as one fiery, self-centered man-of-the-world. His sexual reputation is both that of the promiscuous rogue and the knight in shining armor. He's an idealist about love and sex, a traveler, and opportunist. If you're as independent and enthusiastic as he is, you might be his best friend.

> Mr. Sagittarius thrives on a **light-hearted approach** to life and will take sex **as it comes,** and **as often** as he possibly can

Sounds like just your kind of man? Romantic, sexually dynamic, and hilarious? Well, he is, but he's also a law unto himself. So don't ever treat him as your possession. He needs freedom, and he's a romantic roamer who's liable to have quick flings for the hell of it. However, if you give him enough rope, he usually comes back. Don't believe all that stuff about his exes—most of it is bravado and he does exaggerate. Wild promises about whizzing you off for a weekend in Rome are simply that, and he's not usually able to live up to them. Sagittarius lives in a romantic fantasy world, and that's why commitment is such a terrifying finality for him. So be hilarious, sexy, and Miss Independent to keep him lusting after you.

On a first date, dress simply, and don't dash off to the loo to preen yourself with mascara—he likes the natural look—otherwise the chances are he'll be chatting up someone else by the time you get back. Talk dirty and flirt with his pals to prove you're as carefree, sexually electrifying, and capricious as he is.

HOW TO MAKE HIM HORNY

Not exactly hard. He's permanently on red alert, and if he fancies you, that's enough to put his sex drive on the highest setting. Like the other fire signs, though, he does have a deep-seated fear of sexual inadequacy, which is why he has to compensate by acting the part of the stud that he is. If you want to turn a growing erection into a hot rod, then follow this trick. Tell him you want sex now. Then describe your favorite fantasy with lots of dirty words thrown in between kisses. He finds explicit erotic talk a big turn-on—the naughtier the better! Mr. Sagittarius is not into long, drawn-out foreplay, and he doesn't have time for all that sloppy sensual closeness. After you've got him fired up with your words, surprise him with your uninhibited, upfront approach, unzip his fly and go down on him

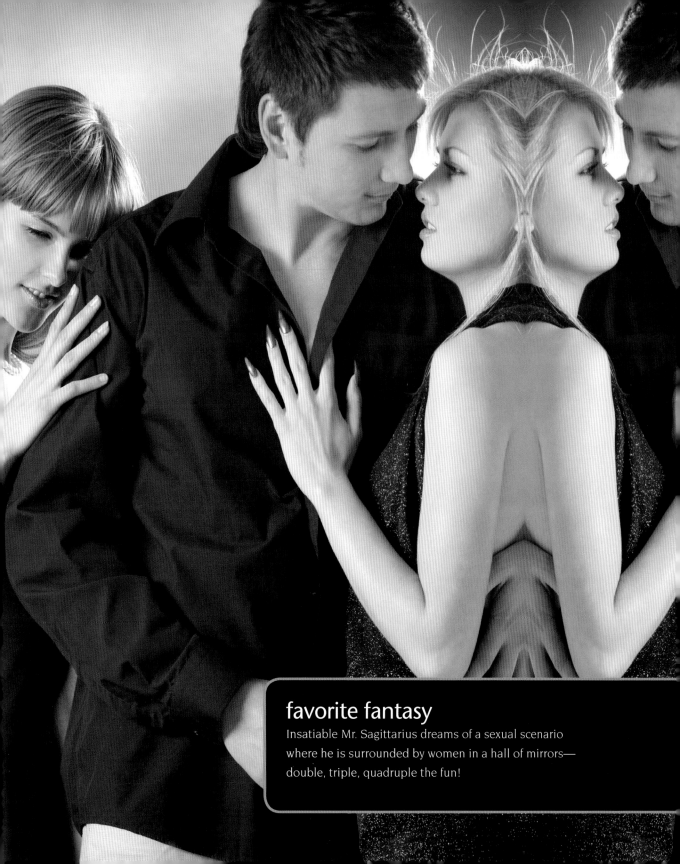

favorite fantasy

Insatiable Mr. Sagittarius dreams of a sexual scenario
where he is surrounded by women in a hall of mirrors—
double, triple, quadruple the fun!

LIVING THE DREAM

Seduce him with tales of your own travels, like how you've had sex with someone famous, like the designer behind Prada's success (not that you can remember his name—it was a quick fling on a press trip). Tell him you're off around the world (even if it's not true, he won't bother to ask why you haven't departed three weeks later) and that you never ever want to be tied down. Then take him outside and have sex. It should do the trick.

RIGHT HERE, RIGHT NOW

Basically, this sexy man is turned on by spontaneous sexual action. Anything from a hand down his trousers when he's driving the car to blindfolding him and licking him all over in the bedroom. Impulsive, unexpected masturbation is a prime arousal trigger. Particularly in public places, where the chance of discovery really gets him horny.

EQUALITY

Once he gets down to the nitty-gritty, Sagittarius likes both to dominate and be submissive. And he's up for role-playing sex too. Pretend you're strangers on a plane, wear saucy underwear one day, dominatrix leather the next, go for a moonlight swim and have sex in the sea, on the beach, in the country, and have wild rampant sex with your clothes on. Indoors (he does have to come inside sometimes), stand behind him in front of a mirror and let him watch you stroke and fondle his penis. He's turned on by your buttocks and hips, so make love doggy-

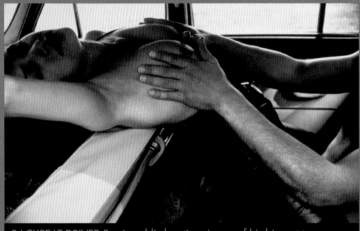

BACKSEAT DRIVER Sex in public locations is one of his biggest turn-ons. Swerve into that lay-by and let him take control.

SWIVEL STICK

Quite honestly, "kama sutra" techniques and sex manuals aren't his style. Don't let him see this book, unless you show him for a laugh! Sex in motion is one of his biggest turn-ons, so try this sequence for variety and movement. Make sure you're fully aroused before attempting this position, as penetration is particularly deep. Lie back on the bed and get him to kneel between your raised legs as he enters you.

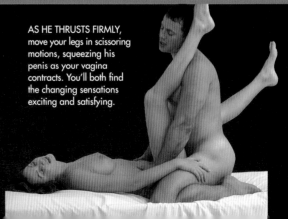

AS HE THRUSTS FIRMLY, move your legs in scissoring motions, squeezing his penis as your vagina contracts. You'll both find the changing sensations exciting and satisfying.

style—in the kitchen, on the stairs, or in the bath.

Talk dirty to him on the phone. Then appear on his doorstep dressed only in a coat or dress, and no underwear. The more daring you are, the greater his sex drive and the more he'll

VARIETY

Sagittarius requires a great deal of sexual variety, which is why he often strays into the arms of a stranger. For him, a different person means different sex: different body, voice, smells, skin—different adventure.

Whether it's a **threesome,** orgy, or **exhibitionist** sex, his imagination knows **no bounds**

want you. He thrives on firm, smooth, and steady rhythms while you masturbate yourself, and he needs to be constantly reassured that his penis really is "the biz." He loves mutual masturbation, followed by sexy pillow fights and intercourse in as many different positions as you can both think up.

But if he's decided you're the one he wants, then he'll be up for marathon sex through the night, unusual locations, and spontaneous oral sex during the day. He'll try anything once, relishes the thought of anal penetration rather the actual experience of it, and gets turned on by his whole fantasy world.

HIS TOP TURNOFFS

COMMITMENT
Suggest that he stays for breakfast after you've had marathon sex and he'll be out of the door before you've turned off the light.

BEING TOLD WHAT TO DO
The free bird won't be caged or ordered around. He'll probably laugh, and then he'll leave you.

RESPONSIBILITY
Don't tell him it's his fault you didn't have an orgasm or that he's responsible for your happiness or that it's his turn to wash the dishes. He'd rather die on the torture rack.

REALITY
Jupiter-born Sagittarius really does think he's pretty omnipotent. Never tell him to "get real": the only reality you'll know is his bags being packed.

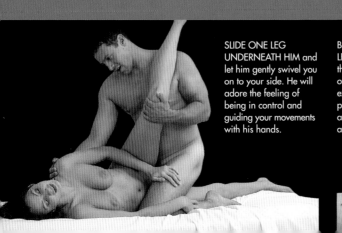

SLIDE ONE LEG UNDERNEATH HIM and let him gently swivel you on to your side. He will adore the feeling of being in control and guiding your movements with his hands.

BRING YOUR OTHER LEG across his body. In this position, the weight of your legs will put exciting pressure on his penis, and his hands are free to caress your abdomen and clitoris.

IS THIS THE ONE?

By now you've probably guessed that idealistic Sagittarians don't find it easy to commit to long-term relationships. They quickly become bored or feel trapped. But there are some signs who can keep them on their toes, for a while.

ARIES AND SAGITTARIUS

All fire and brimstone, to begin with. But when the flames die down, what's left? Probably the desire to go your own way. Sexy, but peppered with electric highs and fiery blow-ups. Can be creative, if both realize you've got hearts as well as egos.

TAURUS AND SAGITTARIUS

Sagittarius loves to feel free and doesn't want commitment; Taurus needs stability. Sexually fascinating, but long-term isn't easy unless Taurus gives Sagittarius all the rope in the world, and the archer comes home occasionally to find out why.

GEMINI AND SAGITTARIUS

A magnetic sexual attraction. Sagittarius leaps into Gemini's life bringing adventure, but can disappear fast. If you don't expect anything from each other, the archer may still be calling Gemini from outer space. Exciting, and often lasting.

CANCER AND SAGITTARIUS

The crab is home-loving, but the archer is not exactly fond of domestic bliss. Great for a sexy fling, but in the long-term Cancer won't like being left alone, and Sagittarius will detest Cancer's clingy ways. A very difficult match.

LEO AND SAGITTARIUS

Great for fun and a madcap, passionate affair. But the archer's a roamer, not a fixture and fitting, while Leo treats Sagittarius like a luxury item. Great for boosting each other's images, but bust-ups likely when you each get led astray by a pretty face.

VIRGO AND SAGITTARIUS

Could prove to be a highly exciting adventure if Virgo can tolerate the archer's unreliability. Virgo's intellectual outlook on life impresses Sagittarius, and sexually you are both adaptable. The downside? Virgo wants order; Sagittarius wants anything but.

Completely **romantic** duo to begin with. And you feel as if you've finally met your **perfect match**. Fun, sexy, and **magical**, but Sagittarius may come to feel **trapped** by all those social **expectations** and Libra's habit of saying "we."

The archer needs to **feel free** to come and go; Scorpio needs to know exactly what the archer's up to. Sexually **exciting** and great for a **short-term fling**, but could turn into a very **torrid** affair. Then Sagittarius is likely to **run** to the hills.

You'll be **drawn** to each other because you see the best of yourselves in each other's eyes. Can be a very long-term **duet**. But you're both likely to be **led astray** by strangers when you want to spread your wings. Dynamic and **sizzling** between the sheets.

Physically **competitive** and deeply erotic. But Capricorns want their **partners** to be the **perfect mates** or business partners. Sagittarians **enjoy the role** if it gets them places, but Capricorn can't handle the archer's **flirtatious** side.

Excellent for a **free-roaming** physical relationship. Both of you need oodles of **space** and don't like emotional scenes. You'll find each other mentally **stimulating** and good for equality and friendship. A **creative** relationship and sexually experimental.

Initially **sexy sparks** will fly. But Pisces is even more **elusive** and unreliable than the archer, so you'll probably keep **missing** each other on those last-minute, **impulsive** dates. Great for sexual **spontaneity** and fun, but difficult for decision making.

LIBRA AND SAGITTARIUS

SCORPIO AND SAGITTARIUS

SAGITTARIUS AND SAGITTARIUS

CAPRICORN AND SAGITTARIUS

AQUARIUS AND SAGITTARIUS

PISCES AND SAGITTARIUS

AND THE WINNER IS...

Sagittarians get on at once with the other fire signs, Leo and Aries, as well as people of their own sign. But Sagittarius places value on friendship and equality as the key to long-term love, whereas Aries delights in being the boss, and Leo in being center stage. Opposite signs always hold a strong fascination, and Gemini thrives on freedom and friendship as much as the archer does. But to keep a Sagittarian intrigued and off-balance for long enough to forge a lasting relationship, it has to be Aquarius

LONG-TERM LOVE WITH SAGITTARIUS

These quixotic heroes and heroines of the zodiac fire quite a few love arrows all over the place before they really settle down with anyone. Long-term love with Sagittarians isn't a piece of cake, but if you can live up to their romantic ideal and never trap them, you might have a chance to befriend the most exciting and fun-filled people you'll ever meet.

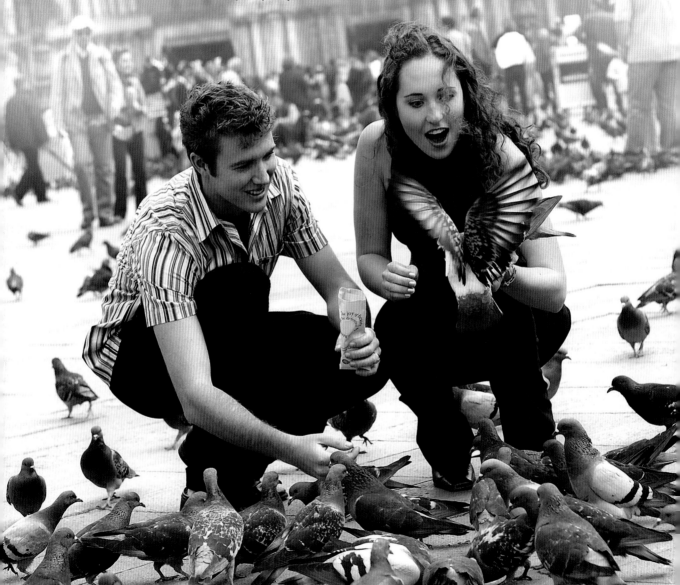

Accept the nomadic, adventurous side of their personality and be prepared for a relationship that gives them enough freedom not to feel tied down: they'll keep coming back for more. Never believe that Sagittarius has no heart. In fact, the archer is a bit of a child, and has a very soft side. The truth is that Sagittarians are so scared of being broken-hearted that they think it's safer to keep moving on from partner to

sometimes crazy plans and throw yourself into everything with energy and joy, you could be their long-term friend and lover. But settling down? Feeling settled for a Sagittarius is to never know where you're going next. So if you're up for an unconventional life, are happy to dash off for a weekend away at the drop of a hat, ready to live in a caravan or trek round the world in search of adventure, then Sagittarius is for you.

HIT THE ROAD

It's incredibly easy to get Sagittarians to dump you. In fact, they'll probably truly believe that they're doing you a favor anyway. Demand a serious commitment, like announcing that it's about time you moved in together, before the archer has even thought beyond the next day, let alone the year ahead. To really get your Sagittarius to hit the road, dump your suitcases in his or her hall and the next you'll hear is a text message from some distant shore: "I've just met this new friend. Thank you for freeing me."

> Archers need to **roam**, whether in their **heads** or on the **road**, and they **need partners** who can **accept** that desire

partner. Show them that you have a heart too, laugh with them, and play with life rather than get serious about it, and they might let you a little bit closer into their worlds. This isn't exactly a stay-at-home sign, so if you prefer sitting in front of the TV or mowing the lawn in suburbia, forget Sagittarius now.

UNCONVENTIONALITY

If you can nurture the archers' dreams, enthuse about their

WANDERLUST

Once you get to the stage in a relationship when a Sagittarian invites you on his or her travels, then you can be pretty sure that he or she wants you as a permanent fixture in his or her flexible life. You could be up for a voyage of a lifetime, but remember: for Sagittarians, long-term love doesn't involve exclusivity or country cottages. It's about freedom first and foremost, friendship second.

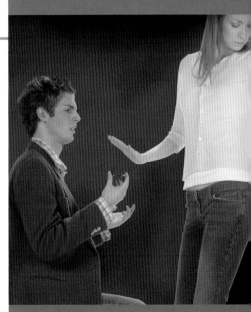

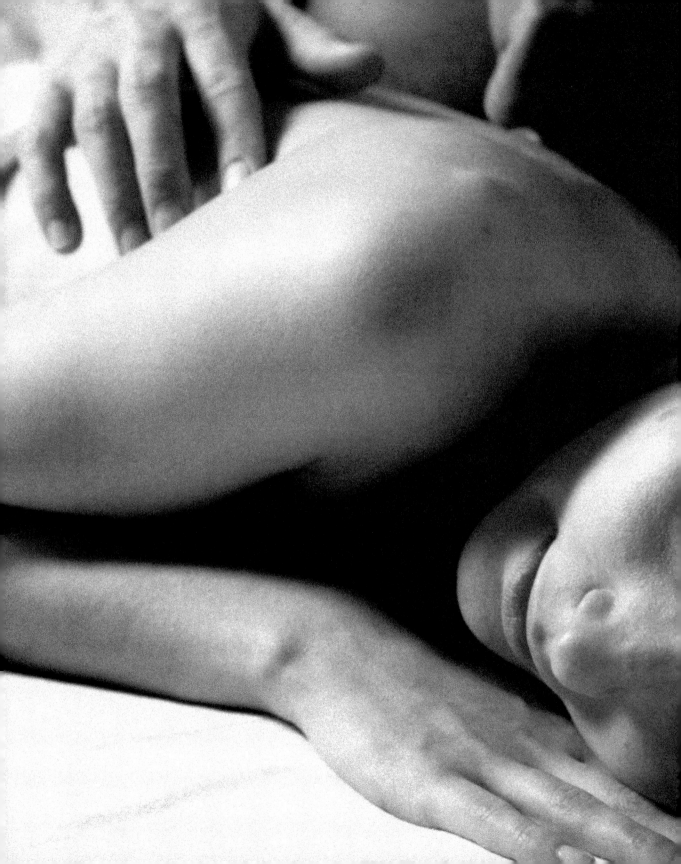

CAPRICORN

DECEMBER 22 – JANUARY 20

STAR STATS

Ruling planet SATURN
Signature symbol THE GOAT
Metal LEAD
Stone BLACK ONYX
Color FOREST GREEN

Where to find Capricorn Music venues, working in big business or the film and music industries.

Hot date Classy restaurant followed by classic "coffee at my place?" Capricorn loves to follow sexual convention.

Needs and desires Down to earth but sensitive, the goat needs closeness, loads of praise, stability, and commitment.

Top turn-on Slow sensual arousal: an aromatherapy body massage surrounded by fragrant candles or low lighting.

Sex positions ♀ The Orchid
♂ The Crab

Sex toy Champagne bubbles.

Sex statistic 83 percent of Capricorns have sex before breakfast, and during it.

WHAT TO EXPECT WITH CAPRICORN

Earthy Capricorn enjoys all the pleasures of the flesh and, like other earth signs, is an utter sensualist when it comes to sex. Cool, classy, and controlling, the goat is ambitious and focused at best, cynical at worst. Capricorns are cautious about forming relationships, but once committed to you, they'll be there for life.

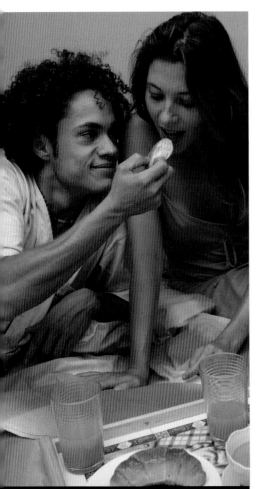

BREAKFAST IN BED The goat likes to start the day with a feast of food and lovemaking.

Capricorn is ruled by Saturn, the taskmaster of the zodiac. And the goat is invariably a seriously motivated sign. Capricorns will work from dusk until midnight to get where they want to be. And similarly, if they fall in love, they'll take as long as it takes to make you theirs. Capricorns don't make a big fuss about seduction. It's passive, careful, and they maintain a detached aura about them, which is simply a shield to protect their acutely vulnerable side. But their sophisticated charisma also exudes an earthy sexuality, and they have the capacity to organize, flirt, play, and work, and still have time to look stunning.

PLAYING BY THE RULES

Accomplished and impeccable, they're conventional about love and sex. When they commit themselves to an intimate relationship, they prefer all the traditional accoutrements—a good home, money in the bank, security, and fidelity. Goats rarely stray, unless of course it means they can rise to the top of their profession.

IN CONTROL

Practical and down to earth, they exude a lush temperament beneath their sometimes shy exteriors. Clock-watchers, they time sex to perfection and will punctually provide you with breakfast in bed every morning. Loyal and dependable, they expect the same in return. They believe in responsibility, duty, and above all the power to run their own lives. Once hooked, they take love deadly seriously. But behind that conventional, aloof ambition lies a secret romantic. They'll probably never admit it, but you'll soon realize that lurking behind the dry sense of humor and mature approach to life is a child who wants to come out and play.

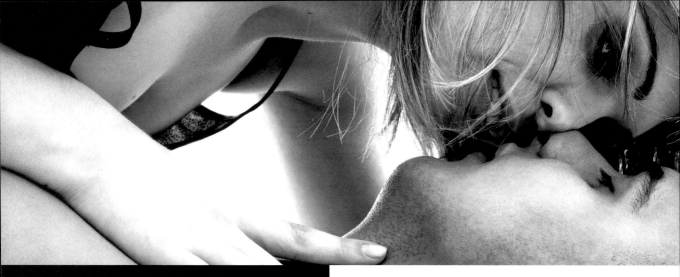

THE CAPRICORN MAN

Mr. Classic-Clothes-and-Clean-Shoes is overtly conventional. He knows what he wants and how he's going to get there. Rugged and realistic, he won't play silly mind games, but he is partial to sports like rugby and power-tripping (nicely) in the bedroom. Emotionally cool, he throbs with manly sexiness. He's seduced by class, beauty, style, expensive tastes, and a woman who knows the difference between claret and burgundy. A bit of a control freak, he's actually quite a soft touch inside, and when he falls for your grace, feminine charm, and brilliant mind, he'll flatter you with roses and take you out for candlelit dinners. In bed, he's sensual, likes to dominate, but also adores you to be on top. If he believes you can be the power behind his throne, he's willing to stick with you through thick or thin. And that could be for life.

THE CAPRICORN WOMAN

Exuding a feral sensuality, classy Miss Capricorn is serious about love and mutual respect. She may appear aloof, but that's because she's hunting for a relationship that really "works." She's secretly

> ## Sex is a commitment, but she might use a fling to get ahead

ambitious in love as well as life, and if you're a professional success, financially solvent, or an older, experienced man then you will be the one she wants. If it takes her ten years to capture your heart, she'll wait. This lady is exactly that: a Lady.

CAPRICORN IN A NUTSHELL

KEYWORDS Self-sufficient; sensual; loyal; cautious; ambitious; highly sexed; traditional; insecure; critical; cool

LIKES Status; security; control; structure; maturity; style; classic clothes and people

DISLIKES Risks; the unknown; radical ideas; dreamers; laziness

TRACKING DOWN YOUR CAPRICORN

Capricorn is a sign who rarely goes off on a tangent. They like the tried and trusted and are certainly easy to track down if you know exactly where to find them. But you've got to have a head for professional or glamorous heights. It's a rare goat who's left stranded at the bottom of the mountain of ambition.

The goat is probably the most ambitious sign of the zodiac, simply because Capricorn's quest for power is fueled by an acute sense of vulnerability. They can and will direct anything from instinct for the pecking order in either the "Establishment" or "glitterazi," and can be found working his or her way up the success ladder in the most glamorous of careers.

> Look for Capricorns in **classy venues**: you're more likely to spot them **onstage** or in the audience at a **recital** than a rave

films to restaurants or galleries. And it is this sense of direction that gets them noticed and gives them the status they crave.

Management, directorship, chairing boards, running a company—all these are within a Capricorn's capacity. Even if they crave family life, they still need to be in a position with a great sense of responsibility. The goat has an extraordinary

SOCIAL CLIMBING

A clock-watcher and timekeeper, Capricorn's a real stickler for routine. So if you're on the track of the goat, you can be sure to find this sign at the same place, same time every day. They can be social climbers in their quest for power and, because they need to feel in control of their lives, Capricorns often end up controlling everyone around

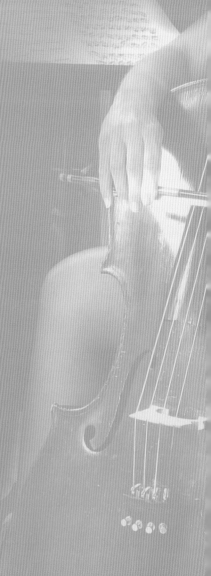

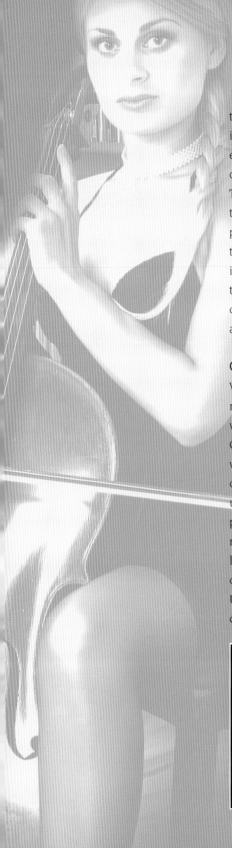

them. It's easy to spot them at important functions or social events: they usually hang out quietly with the star of the show. They rarely make a scene because they really do worry what other people might think of them. And they're sure to be dressed to impress but not stand out from the crowd, nothing flamboyant or flash, just stylish, traditional, and usually expensive.

OUT OF HOURS

Well, goats do need to play more. But finding them out of a work environment isn't too easy. Capricorns often have traditional values. They pitch in a lot at other people's weddings—they usually believe in marriage—and proper dinner parties, and are more likely to pop down to the local bar for a drink than sweat it out in a disco or late-night club. Unless of course, they need to climb that ladder to success.

PLACES TO LOOK

GOURMET RESTAURANTS
Like Taurus, Capricorn is a bit of a connoisseur when it comes to food. And it has to be the best food and finest environment.

CLASSICAL MUSIC CONCERTS
The goat has an innate talent for music. If they're not up on stage as first violin, they'll be attending piano recitals, opening night at the Met or the latest *Carmen*.

JEWELERY SHOPS
A finely cut diamond or a Rolex watch is definitely a Capricorn's best friend. If they're not buying, then they'll be just admiring them.

LUXURY YACHTS
They don't make good sailors, but they love to strut around boat fairs and, of course, lounge about on the deck of their company yacht in any chic marina.

CAPRICORN TOP TEN CAREERS

1	Account executive	6	Celebrity
2	Administrator	7	Diamond cutter/Gemologist
3	Manager	8	Clockmaker/Watchmaker
4	Civil engineer/Property developer	9	Public speaker
5	Government official	10	Geologist

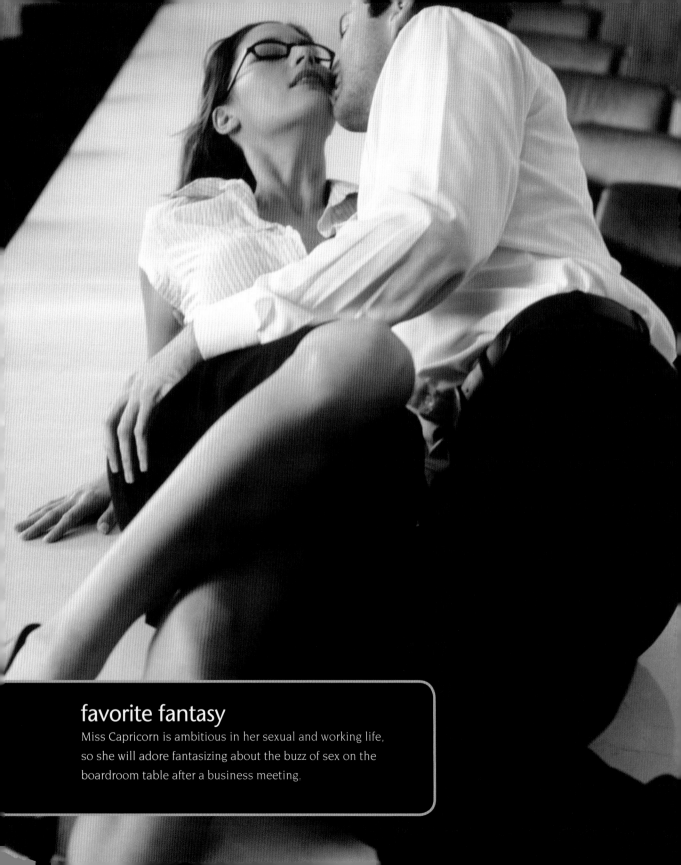

favorite fantasy

Miss Capricorn is ambitious in her sexual and working life,
so she will adore fantasizing about the buzz of sex on the
boardroom table after a business meeting.

WHAT WORKS FOR HER

Sensual but aloof, the Capricorn woman isn't exactly a tigress on the rampage when you first meet her. But behind the coy, polished image that she cultivates she has a high sex drive, and this classy lady can be passion personified if she lets you melt her icy defenses.

Miss Capricorn certainly takes sex seriously, and she makes it her business to be with a man who's got style, class and a steamy sexual style. She prefers conventional types and is often attracted to older men for their wisdom and sexual maturity. The goat's sensual nature is saucy, but she's not usually up for one-night stands. It takes her a long time to trust you, with probably a lengthy string of conventional dates before she'll even suggest coffee at her place, but once she feels safe, her wild side takes over and she can be one of the most

> The Capricorn **lady's** sexuality is **show-stopping** in private, but **aloof** and hidden in public

rampant and wicked women in bed. Power and prestige turn her on, so if you're running for the head of the company or are a bit of a local celebrity, she's more likely to fall for you.

TRUST
The bonding and loving power of sexual pleasure is far more

important to the Capricorn lady than sex for the sake of sex. Discreet and erotic locations enable her to feel aroused, and she needs a skillful lover, who's also earthy and funny. A long-lasting sexual and loving bond is essential for the lady goat, and to orgasm she must have complete affinity with her lover.

HOW TO MAKE HER HORNY

Earthy but cool, sensuous but shy, Miss Capricorn needs time—and lots of it—to get really horny. Massage plays a great part in her arousal pattern. So start by massaging her back, neck, and arms, without aiming straight for more sexual areas like the buttocks or breasts. Use aromatherapy oils or baby oil, and use long, slow strokes of your hands

across her body without stopping. Move up and down her back, spine, and out along her arms, swap to the back of her thighs and knees—her astro-erogenous zone and the epicenter of her sexual-energy flow—and gradually work upward to massage her buttocks while you kiss her shoulders as a sensational taster to foreplay. In the throes of passion, she'll love it if you rub your penis against the back of her knee for ultimate horn-ucopia!

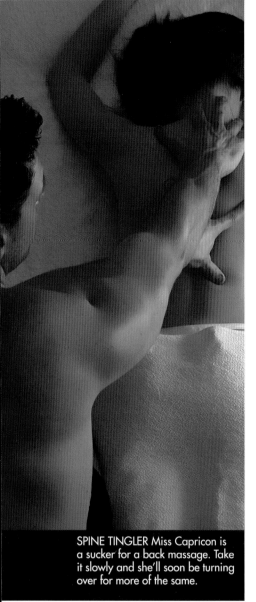

SPINE TINGLER Miss Capricon is a sucker for a back massage. Take it slowly and she'll soon be turning over for more of the same.

HIGH-CLASS RELATIONSHIP

Glamour, success, and material security are all important to Capricorn, and her own career may take up more time than her sex life. Spontaneous sex on a Monday afternoon when she's supposed to be dealing with a work project won't turn her on. Turning off the lights at night will. She thrives on basic, penetrative sex with lots of sensual foreplay, but it has to be at the right time and in the right place, usually indoors, and very private. Ultimately, what this classy, glamorous woman is looking for is a loving, working partnership, not a vague "maybe-see-you-next-week" fling.

SENSUAL BONDING

For maximum arousal, Miss Capricorn needs discretion, skill, and lush arousal. Safety and pleasure are inextricably linked, and she prefers locked doors and sumptuous surroundings to the wild outdoors. Her libido wakes slowly, and you must excel at all the sensual arts to awaken her senses. Massage, wine, and exotic fragrances, a beautiful bed, soft music, and lighting are all favorite accoutrements for Capricorn. Once she feels safe, she becomes a subtle artist of lush sexual domination. She loves to be slowly caressed, her whole body tingling with sensual awareness. Foreplay must be teasing and sultry and she is famous for her extraordinary French-kissing techniques, with oral sex to follow. Because she likes to dominate, she'll prefer to take the lead, her tongue skilled at every delicious move around your penis.

As an earthy, accomplished woman, she craves a close, bonding sex position where

THE ORCHID

Hard, powerful penetration is the joy of this position, with the added bonus for your Capricorn lady that she's on top—something that's sure to please! Being in control maximizes her physical and emotional stimulation, and she'll be more than willing to share the pleasure. Ask her to caress her clitoris and bring herself to peaks of orgasmic energy. Then lie back and let her take over for truly sensational sex.

ORAL SEX SATISFIES HER DESIRE to take the lead, so let her move slinkily down your body to tongue and suck your penis.

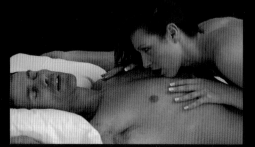

HER TOP TURNOFFS

PENIS BRAINS
Crude behavior or a "slap and tickle" approach to sex will send her running. She needs refined, sophisticated sex, not a gormless wonder who's got his brain on the end of his penis.

AFFECTION IN PUBLIC
Never neck, kiss, or fondle her in public: she really does worry about what other people think when her reputation is at stake.

FLIRTING WITH OTHERS
You must give her your undivided attention or the goat will seek out new pastures.

EMPTY WALLET
You may have the charm of Don Juan, but if you don't have a full wallet or an expense account, her insecurity will be your downfall.

she can express her need to dominate. The Orchid is the perfect sex position for her as it honors her need to feel deeply bound to you, both emotionally and physically.

MISS STRIPTEASE
Miss Capricorn just loves to play different roles, from the stripteasing dancer to the schoolgirl or teacher. In fact, she's a bit of a tease herself once you get to know her intimately, and she'll adore surprising you with tricks and tips she's learned both through her desire to be the most accomplished sexual woman in the world and from all the books and sex manuals she's lined up on her bedside table.

One of her favorite teasing turn-ons is to fall into a scented bath just before you arrive to find her masturbating alone.

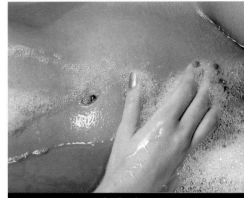

RUB-A-DUB-DUB She'll adore your full attention at bathtime, especially if you give her a helping hand beneath the bubbles.

Wake her up in the morning with your own kind of sexual surprise. She adores being passive and receptive before sex, then turning the tables. Take a bath together and ask her to sit between your legs, her back against your belly. Caress her clitoris and vagina beneath the foam for bubbling arousal. Then let her take control of the action—and your penis.

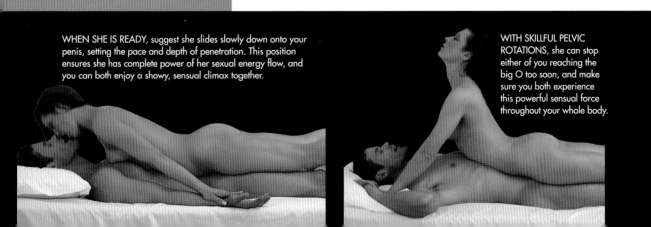

WHEN SHE IS READY, suggest she slides slowly down onto your penis, setting the pace and depth of penetration. This position ensures she has complete power of her sexual energy flow, and you can both enjoy a showy, sensual climax together.

WITH SKILLFUL PELVIC ROTATIONS, she can stop either of you reaching the big O too soon, and make sure you both experience this powerful sensual force throughout your whole body.

WHAT WORKS FOR HIM

Smart but low-key, sensible but carnal, the stylish Capricorn man demands class and grace in the bedroom, and his desire for long-term commitment and ambitious partnerships make him much sought after. He takes a while to warm up, but when he does, his technique and passion are worth the wait.

Capricorn believes he **knows** what's **best for you**—and the **rest of the world**—and funnily enough, he's **usually right**

Control is everything to this earthy, practical man. And you will probably notice that he's shrewdly controlling you on those first dates by looking at his watch, checking the time, planning the next step of the conventional art of seduction.

He does have a tendency to be a bit of a control freak both at the office (ruthlessly) and in bed (nicely). But you always know where you stand with him. You won't get romantic rubbish spouted at you across the restaurant table, only real

tangible ambition while he hopes beyond all hope that you're really up for sexy lingerie, champagne on ice, and slow sensual arousal.

TRADITIONAL VALUES

He's as traditional about love and sex as he is about life. And the goat has a deep-seated sense of responsibility about it all too. If you're having a good time in his company then he'll take it as a sign he's scored some serious brownie points. Then again, if you aren't having an orgasmic time in bed, it's all his fault.

HOW TO MAKE HIM HORNY

Capricorn may like to dominate in bed, but he's certainly up for back scratching, aromatherapy massage, and all the kind of sensual arts that geishas, houris, sex slaves, and you, of course, can provide. Turning him on isn't so much a long, drawn-out affair as a carefully constructed, conventional route to the next stage when he can take over the action. Give

him a sensual back-and-front massage, then follow through with an all-over body massage from the top of his neck down to his ankles to get every inch of him tingling. The back of his knees are his astro-erogenous zone and get more and more sensitive the more aroused he gets. Concentrate on this area with light kisses and licks and then, for the *grande finale*, massage him again all over, but this time with your breasts and nipples.

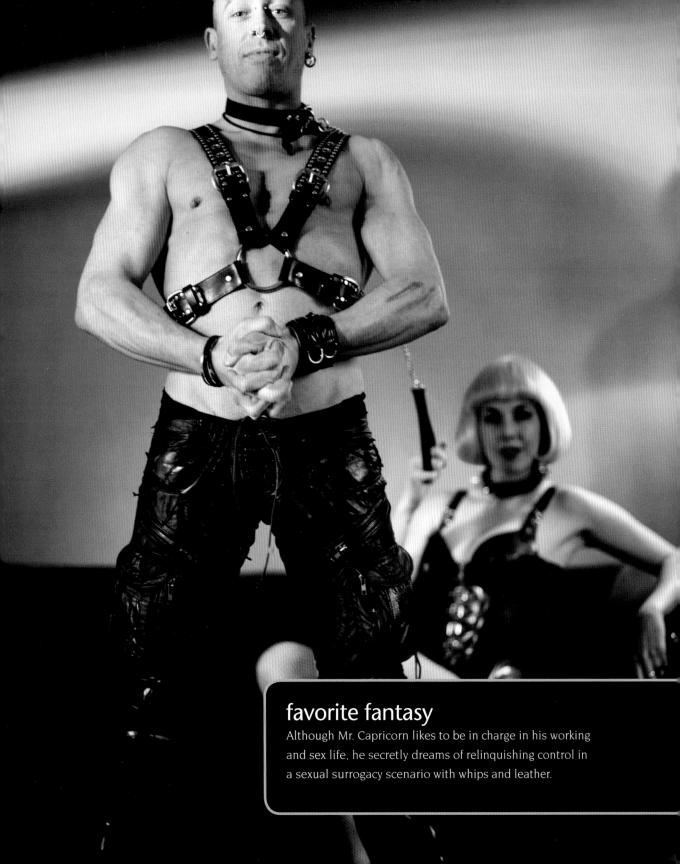

favorite fantasy

Although Mr. Capricorn likes to be in charge in his working and sex life, he secretly dreams of relinquishing control in a sexual surrogacy scenario with whips and leather.

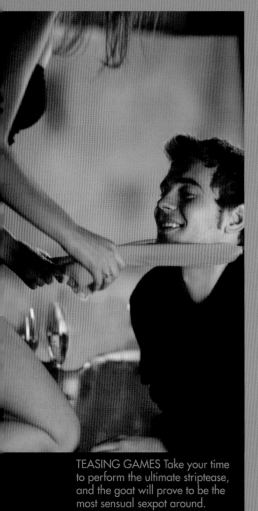

TEASING GAMES Take your time to perform the ultimate striptease, and the goat will prove to be the most sensual sexpot around.

SERIOUS ABOUT YOU

He may not be up for sex in a back alley, and is hardly likely to kiss you in public, but once he thinks you're worthy of his attention, he's likely to hang around longer than most other signs and prove that he's one of the most reliable, masculine, and accomplished of lovers. But for all his self-discipline, style, and ambition, there's a child behind the mask who desperately needs to come out to play. Be his sexual playmate and you'll probably become the power behind his throne too.

AMBIENCE

Romantic locations, subtle lighting, beautiful fragrance, the way you wear your clothes and undress will keep Capricorn turned on for hours. Just by virtue of being a truly sensual woman, you'll have little trouble seducing him to your ways. But be straight down the line, frank, and honest about your sexual needs. Remember, he does take responsibility for how you feel too. A pillar of strength may be a little clichéd, but he's certainly able to play a towering inferno of passion when it suits him.

The goat needs to feel in control in the bedroom, and doesn't like to be hurried. He has a fairly consistent pattern of arousal each time he makes love. However, he is quickly aroused by suggestive but discreet sex talk in private. The more alluring and feminine you are, the better. Perform a striptease when you are alone at home, slowly and sensually, and remember he's turned on by the ambience of the occasion—moody, sultry low lighting, chilled wine to sip while he watches you, and sexy music to make love to.

THE CRAB

This man adores being on top most of the time. Classic lovemaking, like the Missionary position, satisfies his desire for control and deep penetration. The Crab, with its exciting visuals and male dominance, is perfect to get his libido racing. Once he's aroused, he'll also love you to take a turn on top: he's especially turned on by the sight of your exposed clitoris as you lean back.

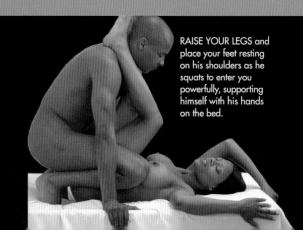

RAISE YOUR LEGS and place your feet resting on his shoulders as he squats to enter you powerfully, supporting himself with his hands on the bed.

STRAIGHTFORWARD

The goat is hardly a Casanova, although in his early youth he might play around simply to get enough experience and become accomplished in every sexual way. He quite likes sex books, manuals, videos, and the odd

Power and domination give him the biggest adrenaline surge, so beg him for sex and then let him rip your clothes off. Smear each other in baby oil, and he'll be instantly aroused for a slippery love session. Stroke, caress, and tease his inner thighs during

> He is into **straightforward** sex, although he may **fantasize** about **experimenting**

bit of porn. But he's a meat and potatoes man, and experimental sexual relationships or S&M just can't beat straightforward, hard penetration and some oral sex thrown in for fun.

AROUSING ANTICS

Run your tongue around his belly button to send him all gooey.

foreplay and he'll be eager for the 69 position. His buttocks are prime sexual triggers, so bite them playfully, or quite hard if you like—he's secretly fond of a bit of rough and tumble. Rub your breasts across his penis and bring yourself to orgasm while you do so: he adores the thrill of seeing you climax.

HIS TOP TURN OFFS

FLIRTATIOUSNESS

He hates being embarrassed in public and worries what other people think of him. Keep the sauce strictly for him, in the privacy of the bedroom.

BEING LATE

You must be as punctual as the goat: time waits for no woman.

IMMATURITY

He's looking for someone who is self-motivated and serious, mature and wise. Any childish behavior in public will drive him crazy.

FLASH WOMEN

He can't bear women baring breasts and bums in public. And if you're the glitzy type with cheap jewelery dripping off every limb, then forget it. Now one diamond ring, that's another matter.

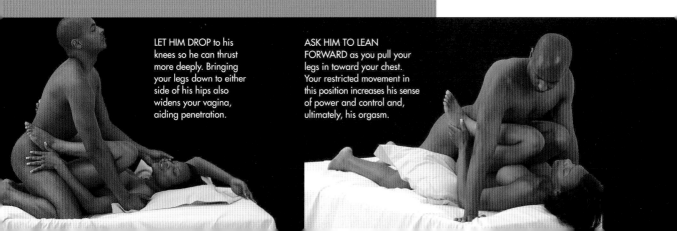

LET HIM DROP to his knees so he can thrust more deeply. Bringing your legs down to either side of his hips also widens your vagina, aiding penetration.

ASK HIM TO LEAN FORWARD as you pull your legs in toward your chest. Your restricted movement in this position increases his sense of power and control and, ultimately, his orgasm.

IS THIS THE ONE?

When it comes to long-term relationships, Capricorn's strength, integrity, and loyalty sets the goats apart from the romance crowd, and their compatibility rating is excellent. But which signs can live up to their ideal?

ARIES AND CAPRICORN

A battle of wills, but a very physical magnetism between you. The ram's egotistical and sometimes thinks the goat's too self-absorbed and serious. But great for a professionally dynamic partnership with loads of sex thrown in.

TAURUS AND CAPRICORN

Sexually perfect. Materially and mentally you're in tune, but you could end up in more fights than you imagine simply because you both get obsessed about who's in control. Mutual success, if you keep cool heads and stay hot between the sheets.

GEMINI AND CAPRICORN

Very different attitudes to sex and life. Steamingly sexy to begin with, but Geminis need constant change in their lives, Capricorns need constancy. Not easy long-term, but could lighten up the goat in the short-term.

CANCER AND CAPRICORN

Opposites in the zodiac always attract. Very sexy rapport, extremely serious, and often highly successful. Takes a while to break through each other's defensive boundaries, but once you've proved you're there for life, you probably will be.

LEO AND CAPRICORN

Exciting, dramatic, and glamorous, this strangely makes for a steamy relationship. Capricorn loves Leo's sexual style; the lion adores the goat's potent, earthy libido. Problems arise as you both need to dominate in and out of the bedroom.

VIRGO AND CAPRICORN

You have an affinity for the same pleasures in life. A sexually fulfilling relationship, as Virgo understands Capricorn's need for power and prestige. As long as the goat puts up with Virgo's mercurial, teasing side, could be a smash hit.

Very **different approaches** to sex and life. Capricorn thrives on straightforward, **no-nonsense** relationships. Libra is a **romantic** and believes there's always someone better around the corner. **Sexually sizzling**, but usually short-lived.

LIBRA AND CAPRICORN

Challenging and often highly successful. You're both driven by **power**, and both prefer a **private** relationship. The only downside is that Capricorn's a bit of a **social climber**, and Scorpio could get **jealous**. Sexually great, emotionally exhausting.

SCORPIO AND CAPRICORN

Makes for a **physically competitive** relationship, and you are **fascinated** by each other's differences. But Sagittarius hates feeling that **"this is it,"** and the goat won't be able to handle the archer's **flirtatious** nature.

SAGITTARIUS AND CAPRICORN

Sexy rapport, but although you both understand the other inside out, you always feel there's something **missing**. Power-plays and **rivalry** likely, but one of you might fall in love with a **wild romantic** while the other's being **head-hunted**.

CAPRICORN AND CAPRICORN

Different needs, as the goat is **conventional**, and Aquarius is **anything but**. A lively, demanding, and **ambitious** rapport, as long as Capricorn gives Aquarius some **space** and Aquarius gives the goat the time of day. Better for **working** than sex.

AQUARIUS AND CAPRICORN

Pisces' **changeable moods** makes the goat uncomfortable. Not an easy rapport, as Capricorn wants things to be **black and white** while Pisces prefers a few **grey areas**. You could fall head over heels in love but regret it later. **Sexy** but **unstable**.

PISCES AND CAPRICORN

AND THE WINNER IS...

Well, being the ultimate lover of long-term relationships, the goat is ideally suited to both Taurus and Virgo and is likely to have a sexy and long-lasting rapport with Aries, Cancer, and Scorpio. But if you have to pick just one winner, then secure and sensual Taurus is probably the outright champion. Not only do both signs have the same sexual desires and responses but they're both driven to achieve in the outer world and have an affinity for material security.

LONG-TERM LOVE WITH CAPRICORN

Marriage, fidelity, and vows suit Capricorn, eventually. In fact, the goat places great value on long-term love, mutual respect, and the building up of a secure, safe foundation between two people. Yet Capricorn can take forever to do so. If you want a serious commitment, then this is the sign for you. However, if you're an individualist who'd rather play with fire or yearn for never-ending romance, then stay away.

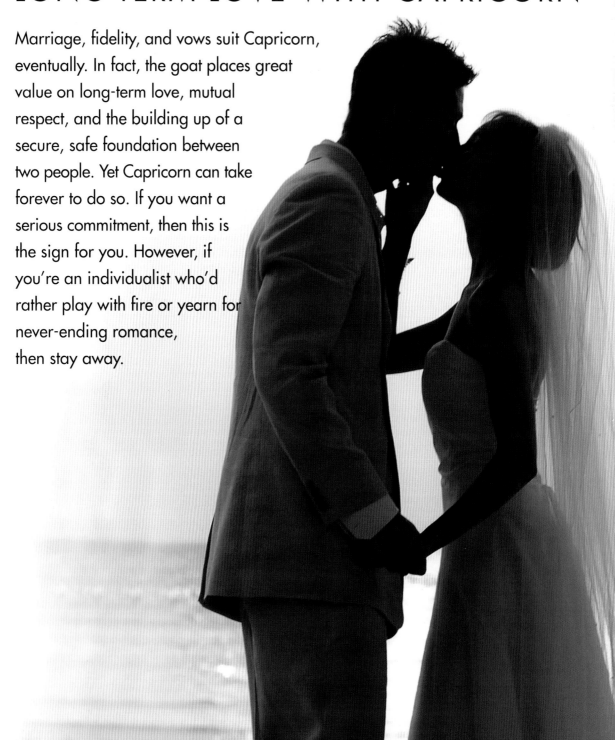

Capricorns admire success, and when they finally decide to mate for life, it's usually with someone who is just as classy, strong-minded, and ambitious for the goat as they are for themselves. They will be your pillar of strength, but in return you must show utter devotion and appreciation of their need for stylish living and an uncluttered and orderly home and be willing to be the secret power behind their throne.

they make a mistake? But if you are down to earth, understand convention and traditional role-playing, are as sensually indulgent as they are, and believe like the goat that career comes first, the rest second, then you've probably met a match for life.

MY WAY

Capricorns are determined to have everything their way, and their playful spirit usually gets

> Once they accept your **motives** are the **same as theirs,** you can **get on** with the **serious business** of lasting partnership

BIG MATCH

Capricorns admire success and want partners who are as driven as they are. However, they can be too calculating in love, simply because they are so insecure and need to feel in control of the heartstrings. Prove that you are trustworthy and can be let out at night without flirting with everyone. Capricorns are terribly cautious about making the "big" commitment, because what if

firmly squished out of any love relationship once they've gone beyond the "dating" stage. But they do need to play as well, otherwise you get bossy goats who will want to control not only themselves but your orgasm, your work, and your mutual future. Or if you're lucky, you'll find a Capricorn who wants to aim for the top, with you at his or her side. Goats need to learn to let go and trust a little.

ESCAPE-GOAT

What Saturn-ruled Capricorns detest above all things is erratic behavior and poor timekeeping. So if you're up for a sly way to get on the wrong side of Capricorn so your goat will chuck you, be totally undependable. Turn up late when you're supposed to be meeting up, make sure you are never available on the phone, and always change your mind at the last minute. Make a firm date and then call to cancel it— half an hour after you were due to be there. It won't be long (and a Capricorn will probably time it to the second) before your goat will make a great escape.

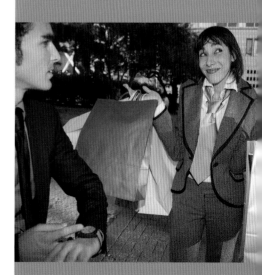

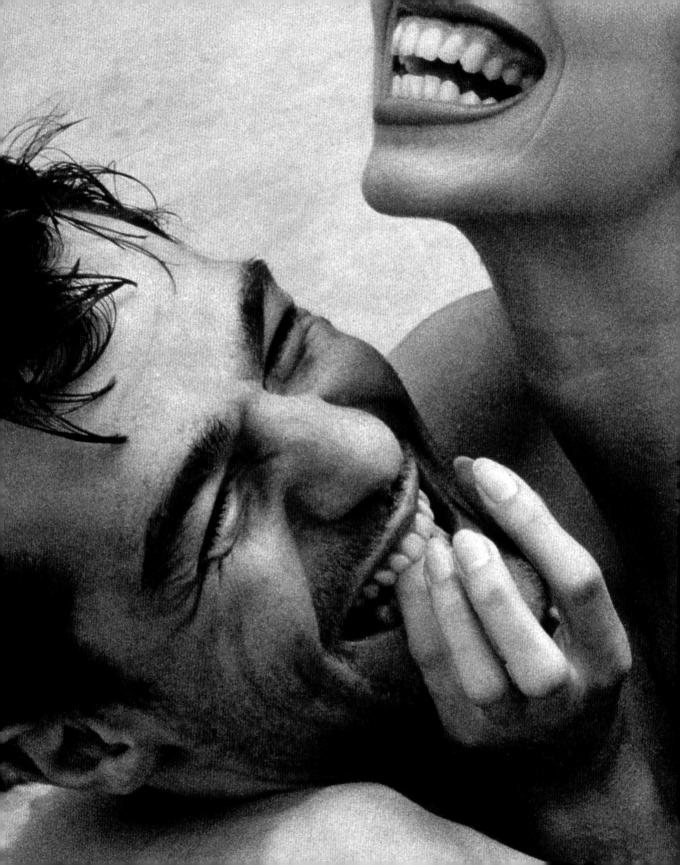

AQUARIUS
JANUARY 21 – FEBRUARY 18

STAR STATS

Ruling planet URANUS
Signature symbol THE WATER-BEARER
Metal ALUMINIUM
Stone LAPIS LAZULI
Color ULTRAMARINE

Where to find Aquarius Working in hi-tech jobs, saving whales, leading protest marches, or visiting safari parks.

Hot date Take Aquarius to see a sci-fi or humanitarian documentary film, then discuss life over a bottle of organic wine.

Needs and desires Original, romantic, and zany, Aquarius needs plenty of space, freedom, and a lover who's not after a conventional relationship.

Top turn-on Unpredictable sex, now—anywhere you happen to be, like the kitchen table.

Sex positions The Maverick
 Pick and Mix

Sex toy Alien masks.

Sex statistic 91 percent of Aquarians are up for bisexual relations.

WHAT TO EXPECT WITH AQUARIUS

Intellectual, avant-garde, and freedom-loving, Aquarians are sexually broad-minded. They are quirky in their taste of lover and prefer to talk about you as a "friend" rather than a partner. Emotional commitment brings them out in spots, but if you're as independent as they are, you could have a friend for life.

Unpredictable Uranus rules Aquarius, and the water-bearers' unconventional lifestyle says a lot about their sexual needs too. If you're looking for an intelligent but noncommittal relationship, then they'll be happy to oblige. However, Aquarius is not good on feelings. In fact, Aquarians may have an awful lot to say about human nature—their psychological observations of sexual deviants are fascinating—but they tend to squish all feelings in favor of the mind.

INDEPENDENT
Aquarians keep a certain distance. They have a dreadful hang-up about intimacy. OK, sex is one thing if they can analyze why they're doing it—to have pleasure or fun, to show off their latest technique, to prove they're "different"—but to feel physically close, contained, or emotionally involved in sex is terrifying to them. Aquarians are really seeking a friend first, sex later. And it's not that they're "unsexy" or have problems with orgasms, it's just they want to keep it all clinical and unmessy. In fact, they're sexually experimental and love shocking you with their bizarre antics and progressive ideas. The water-bearers often act as if they don't give a hoot about sexual passion, but deep down they really would like to be head-over-heels in love like the rest of the human race—they just can't bear all the stuff that goes with it. However, if you're independent and can discuss the universe and everything in it from a rational, objective viewpoint, then maybe—just maybe—you will form a special long-lasting bond.

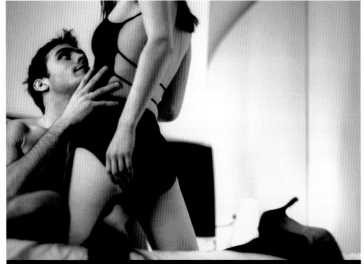

UNPREDICTABLE Aquarians will constantly surprise you with their flair for erotic body language laced with intelligent chitchat.

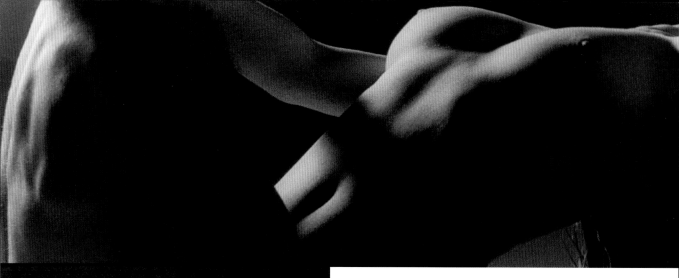

THE AQUARIUS MAN

He's turned on by what's going on in your mind rather than your perfume, cleavage, or feminine behavior. He finds overtly sexual gestures threatening, but if you're unconventional and

Don't **assume** that you know when he's horny: he's one step ahead

clearly have no intention of depending on him, then you might make a first date. He has as many female friends as he does male and is probably in touch with his exes. He's hard to read, with a complex sex drive: just when you think he's not interested, he probably is, and vice versa.

THE AQUARIUS WOMAN

Miss Independent craves the unpredictable and the unusual. She is quite capable of separating sex from love, because the sex gives her freedom while love tends to imply commitment and emotional intimacy. However, that doesn't mean she's promiscuous, only that she's not going to fall for the same old conventional equation that romance plus sex equals love and marriage. Her sexual opinions about threesomes, group sex, and bisexuality are progressive, but she rarely ends up acting on those beliefs. It's not that she's a prude, just that she's happier hiding behind an intellectual safety curtain—the idea is safer than the reality. Remove the curtain at your peril. But if you can be the wittiest, most intelligent, independent, and altruistic man about town, and give her bags of freedom too, she might just begin to let you come a little closer. And this woman is interesting close up.

AQUARIUS IN A NUTSHELL

KEYWORDS Quirky; aloof; avant-garde; independent; intellectual; glamorous; truthful; idealistic

LIKES Personal freedom; human and animal rights; intelligence; minimalist or "green" lifestyles; discussing sex

DISLIKES Emotions; marriage; possessiveness; weepy films

TRACKING DOWN YOUR AQUARIUS

Intellectually driven, the water-bearer is motivated by the welfare of the world rather than individuals. It's not so hard tracking them down if you're up for human rights, education, or hi-tech knowledge. The problem is, unless you're as smart as they are, you'll be just another face in the crowd.

However, if you're bright, shrewd, and can talk about anything from nuclear physics to abortion issues without flinching, then they might take you up on a personal date. Whether an

to suit whatever's going to be the next flavor of the month.

EVERYONE'S FRIEND
Aquarians are ready to crusade for causes that they personally

Whether chatting **online** or researching their latest **arcane interest**, the one with the laptop is probably an **Aquarian**

astrophysicist or a psychologist, Aquarians are likely to be found investigating radical systems or discovering universal truths. Forward-thinking, they make excellent scientists, educators, or fashion gurus. Ultimately they need a consuming passion for something to take them to the top of the tree. But, intuitively, they tap into the future and tailor their professional lifestyles

believe in—anything from persuading shoe manufacturers to stop using leather to finding water on Mars. And if you have as much zeal for a mission as they do, then they might just consider you worth getting to know. It's great that they believe that love makes the world go round, but if you're trying to seduce an Aquarian, remember that they treat everyone as their best friend. In fact, intimate one-to-one relationships are very hard for the Aquarian's non-exclusive perception of love.

EXPECT THE UNEXPECTED

It's pretty hard keeping up with Aquarians both in their working and social lives. One day they're passionate about going to that VIP party to make contacts, the next they'd rather stay in and read that book about social anthropology. They're often found where you least expect them to be, simply because they like being awkward. You'll bump into them on most social occasions. And for all their "let's save the whale" progressive thinking, they're actually social climbers who like to mingle with jet-setters, politicians, celebrities, and academics. That's where they can upset the applecart with their zany ideas and set a new trend of thought.

PLACES TO LOOK

HUMAN RIGHTS PROTESTS
Probably carrying the flag for whatever they believe in. They like to make it clear where their loyalties lie. You'd better too.

HEALTH-FOOD SHOPS
Anything vegetarian goes in the Aquarian book. So give up meat and hang around organic restaurants, delicatessens, and health-food shops.

INTERNET CAFES
Aquarians can't stay away from their technology fix however far they travel. You'll often spot them tapping away on laptops or their cell phone in the middle of a crowd.

FASHION SHOWS
If they're not showing off their latest collection, you can be sure they're the ones who are three seasons ahead of everyone else.

AQUARIUS TOP TEN CAREERS

1	Scientist	6	Educational advisor
2	Hi-tech whiz kid	7	Psychologist
3	Dealer in futures	8	Ecologist
4	Humanitarian reformer	9	Inventor
5	Fashion designer/Trendsetter	10	Astrologer

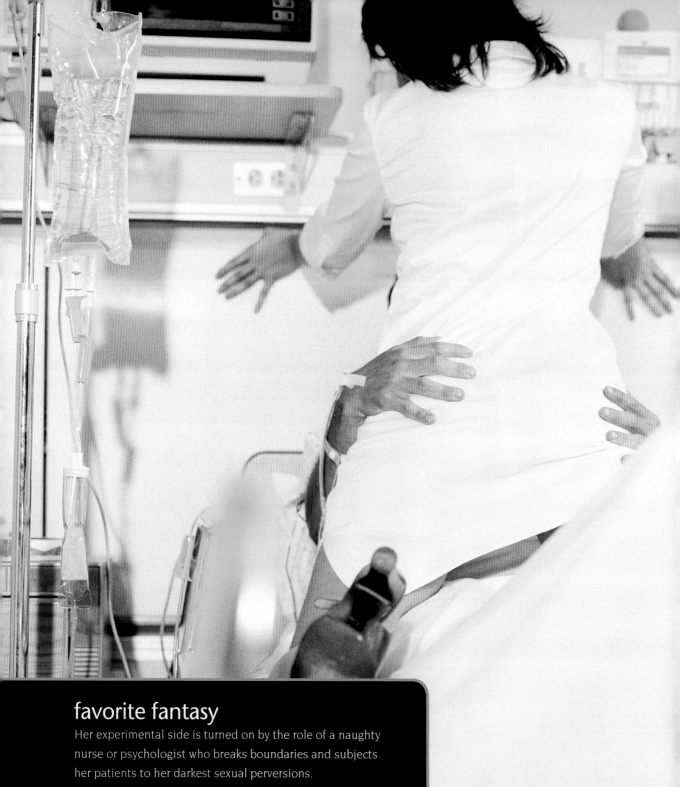

favorite fantasy

Her experimental side is turned on by the role of a naughty
nurse or psychologist who breaks boundaries and subjects
her patients to her darkest sexual perversions.

WHAT WORKS FOR HER

Enigmatic Miss Aquarius is a cool customer. She's seeking a friend first, and a sexual partner comes a long way second. However, if she does get turned on by your mind, then she's going to be the most radical, experimental, and shocking woman you can find in the bedroom.

In fact, Aquarius thinks she ought to try out everything, from anal sex to S&M. A part of her wants to liberate herself from conventional assumptions about what sex "ought to be." However, when she does get involved in "alternative" sexual relationships, she then flips to wanting the conventional "one man, one woman" type again.

The Aquarian woman has a habit of deliberately asking for sex in the most embarrassing places, anywhere that gets her noticed as being utterly different, and she often gets involved in

> If you're a **mystery** man and can offer **unusual** techniques and **erotic** conversation, you'll keep this unique woman **fascinated**

lesbian relationships just to shock friends or family. However, once she's discovered and fully analyzed everything there is to know about your sexual habits, intellect, and psychological makeup, she can get bored and turn off like a light.

FOLLOW MY LEADER

Sexually, Miss Aquarius likes to take the lead and think up exotic ways to orgasm. Her arousal is unique and self-possessed, and you must honor her emotional detachment and joy in physical sex rather than deeper intimacy.

HOW TO MAKE HER HORNY

Aquarius is aroused by erotic chitchat. In fact, she's more likely to prefer talking about sex all night before she actually gets around to doing it. Dominating and unpredictable, she gets off on being in control. So make sure you talk about all the things you want to do with her, and follow her verbal lead. But to prove you're one jump ahead in

the physical stakes, the epicenter of the Aquarian sexual energy flow exudes from her ankles. Caress or massage this potent astro-erogenous zone with your fingers, lips, or tongue, then run your tongue slowly up her legs, along her inner thigh and back down again. Follow this up by tweaking her nipples, rubbing and playing with them while you go down her—oral sex is one of her greatest turn-ons and frees her up from any inhibitions.

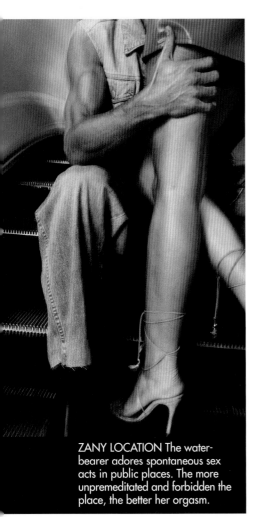

ZANY LOCATION The water-bearer adores spontaneous sex acts in public places. The more unpremeditated and forbidden the place, the better her orgasm.

EXOTIC

For all her cool and aloof ways, Aquarius has a powerful sex drive, and the more she talks sex the more aroused she gets. She needs a lover who responds to her zany, unpredictable sexual style. This woman likes to take control and also to play different roles. Aroused quickly by oral sex, she prefers to be on top rather than be submissive. Orgasm is a cosmic and mind-expanding experience for her. Mutual masturbation ensures she can act as the catalyst for your potent and mind-blowing pleasure, as well as her own.

One of her greatest sexual triggers is spontaneous oral sex in a bizarre location. Like in the car of a Ferris wheel or in the bathroom of a train or plane. Phone her at unexpected times of day and tell her your favorite fantasy in graphic detail. When you meet later, ask her to do exactly what you suggested over the phone, however way-out it seems. She's also turned on by the idea of voyeurism, so make sure you have sex in daylight and quickies in the lay-by or behind a tree.

MIND GAMES

Miss Aquarius's sexual expression is glamorous and avant-garde on the surface. Intellectual arousal is a must and she's curious to experiment with all kinds of sexual foreplay, both in her mind and in your bed. She's probably cornered the market for sexual experimentation by the time she's in her twenties, and she'll lick, dominate, submit, and shock, simply because she's aroused by watching you have fun too. But the one secret about Miss Aquarius is that, for all her sexual know-how, mind-blowing orgasms, and experimentation

THE MAVERICK

The exchange of sexual energy in this position is coextensive, which is essential for her own sense of equality. Although you are controlling her leg movements, she can set a rhythm by squeezing her vaginal muscles, and will let you know verbally exactly what speed and pressure she enjoys. The Maverick enables her to indulge in raw physical energy, while intoxicating you with her wild, unpredictable climaxes.

KNEEL ON THE BED and ask her to raise her legs while you enter her. Kiss and caress her ankles—her astro-erogenous zone—to make her tingle with pleasure.

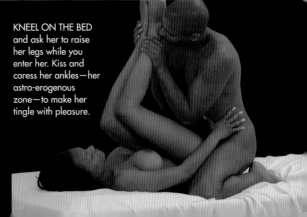

HER TOP TURNOFFS

NAIVE IDIOTS
She can't bear conventional, God-fearing mama's boys, who haven't ever seen a "Jessica Rabbit" or think love eggs are something given at Easter.

COMMITMENT
Words like "marriage," "my woman," "us" or "my partner" bring her out in spots. She's autonomous and you'd better accept it.

THE ORDINARY
The Missionary position, lights off, and vague gropings in the dark are definite no-go areas. She wants to explore the new and daring.

FEELINGS
Never ask her how she feels, only what she thinks. This unconventional woman is primed to love from her head, not her heart.

she's quite inhibited about truly merging in sexual union. You'll notice that after she orgasms she usually goes cold, won't particularly want to be held in a tender embrace, and finds it hard to give affection and warmth. Sex doesn't mean tenderness and bonding to this woman. She fears intimacy and showing her real feelings, so sex is often just for pleasure. That doesn't mean she's an easy lay, but it does mean there's always the nagging feeling that you don't really know who you are really with.

TRY ANYTHING ONCE
Seeing as she's a broad-minded, independent, and experimental Aquarian, she'll try all kinds of kinky sex positions. It gives her a powerful thrill to try out anything acrobatic because it means she doesn't have to get

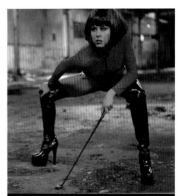

PLAYTIME Kinky is a word probably invented for Miss Aquarius. Get the sex toys out and let the games commence!

too involved in a heated exchange of passion and lets her control her own multiple orgasms. She adores sex where she can analyze your moves, think ahead, and be ready to change roles or positions when it suits her. Unpredictable and energetic, Miss Aquarius is up for all the latest sex toys and gadgets, and will love to play out extreme sexual roles.

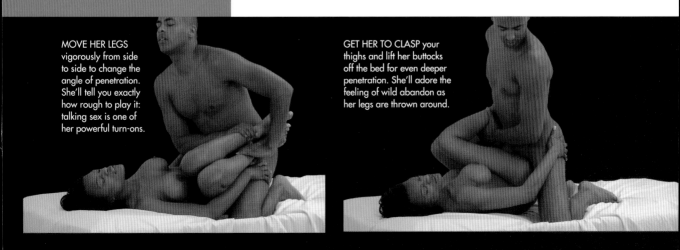

MOVE HER LEGS vigorously from side to side to change the angle of penetration. She'll tell you exactly how rough to play it: talking sex is one of her powerful turn-ons.

GET HER TO CLASP your thighs and lift her buttocks off the bed for even deeper penetration. She'll adore the feeling of wild abandon as her legs are thrown around.

WHAT WORKS FOR HIM

Mr. Aquarius is after sophisticated sex laced with intellectual stimulation. He enjoys analyzing everyone's sexual behavior, so be ready for experimentation and the bizarre. He may not be interested in commitment or emotional intimacy, but he's the most technically original sign of the zodiac, and a true friend.

> You'll never know quite **where you are** with Mr. Aquarius, but if you can **keep up**, you'll be in for an **exhilarating** ride

Mr. Aquarius may seem rather reserved and sexually cool when you first meet him, but he's turned on by your mind first, your body second. If you want to seduce him, start by proving you're as independent as he is, and have as many friends as he does—of both sexes. With a rather erratic libido, when you are convinced he's up for a night out on the town, he wants to stay in and have sex in the kitchen. He likes to be different, experiment, and stand out from his pals. He's not your normal macho type who wants to whirl you around in the bedroom for all-night romps.

INTELLIGENCE

The kind of sex marathons he wants are conversational ones. Teasing erotic language gets him going and he's a sucker for analyzing every move you make. But his is a complex sex drive. If you want to egg him on to go lap-dancing, he'll be there. But make sure he thinks it's his idea. His performance is zany, and often shockingly experimental, so enjoy the unpredictable.

HOW TO MAKE HIM HORNY

Aquarius gets turned on primarily by the erotic thoughts in his mind. He's not that bothered about sensual stuff and foreplay—yes, he'll kiss you like he's put a snake down your throat, but he's not up for steamy, sweaty closeness. On the other hand, he does have a thing for talking about sex, so the quickest way to get him aroused is with a little raunchy chat. Get him rising to attention with plenty of dirty talk while you slide your foot up and down the inside of his thigh (Mr. Aquarius's astro-erogenous zone). Describe your wildest fantasies and exactly what you want to do with him to really get that agile brain of his buzzing. Then reveal your favorite dildo and play dirty with it in front of him. Before you know it, he'll be taking firm control of his extraordinary penis power.

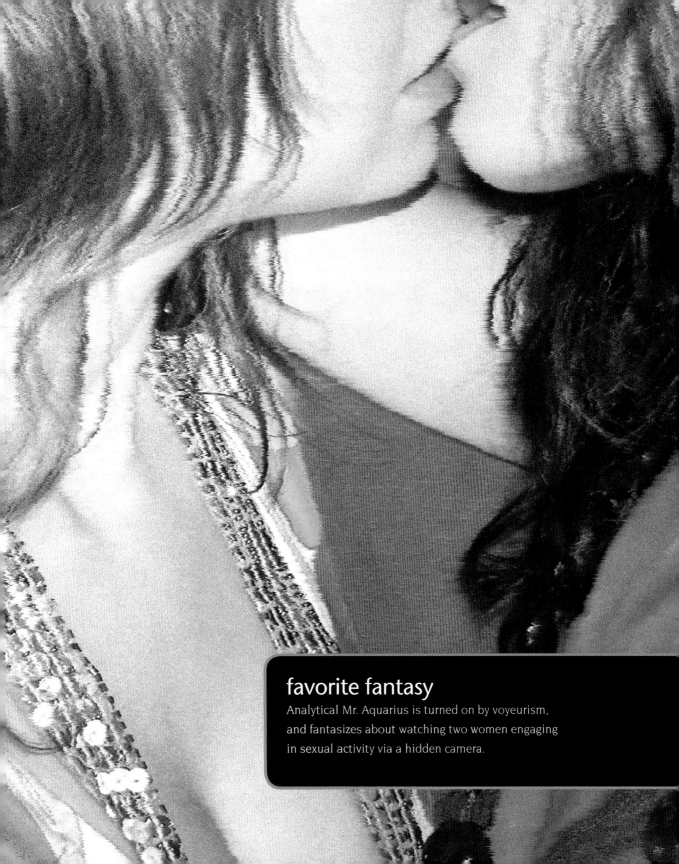

favorite fantasy

Analytical Mr. Aquarius is turned on by voyeurism,
and fantasizes about watching two women engaging
in sexual activity via a hidden camera.

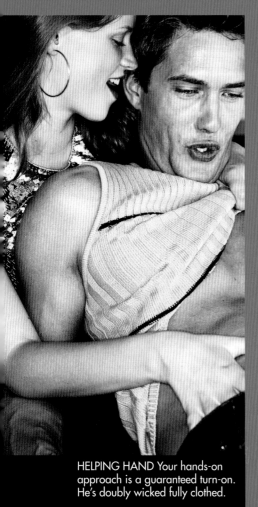

HELPING HAND Your hands-on approach is a guaranteed turn-on. He's doubly wicked fully clothed.

THE UNPREDICTABLE

To keep him hooked, always do the unexpected. If he thinks you're in the mood for sex, tell him he's got to wait until later. If he thinks he's got to wait, seduce him on the floor. Carry on being your fashion-conscious and ahead-of-the-time self. He'll adore you for your ability to accept his eccentric ways and his amazing capacity to think up new ways to have sex. Standing on your head might not be the easiest sex position in the world, but using your head is.

GREAT EXPECTATIONS

He has high expectations of the women he chooses to share his sexual experiences with. If you're already his friend, it's a good start: he likes to feel you're on an equal basis, which is one of his biggest erotic triggers, and aims for simultaneous arousal.

He also likes to switch between dominant and submissive roles.

OUTWARD BOUND

Oral sex is a must, and so is masturbation. Anywhere, and at any time of day. Masturbate him, then sit astride and let him enter you while you're still wearing your clothes. His ultimate turn-on is suggesting sex in unusual or social places. At parties, lure him into the bathroom and make love standing up in front of the mirror. Describe everything you're going to do to him and what you want him to do to you.

He's turned on by surprises. So if you're out on a walk, in a library, or having dinner with friends, whisper in his ear that you want sex now. Then do it.

EROTIC FANTASIES

His mind is a veritable cauldron

PICK AND MIX

Mr. Aquarius has got some funny ideas about sex positions. You don't have to be a gymnast, but he'll adore it if you change angles and positions during sex—the variety of sensations and visuals really turns him on. This sequence gives him the visual and sensual stimulation he gets off on. He'll soon be thinking up new positions to drive you wild.

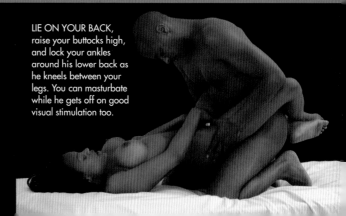

LIE ON YOUR BACK, raise your buttocks high, and lock your ankles around his lower back as he kneels between your legs. You can masturbate while he gets off on good visual stimulation too.

of erotic thoughts. In fact, he'd probably rather tell you all his deepest erotic fantasies while masturbating than be worrying about whether you're coming when he penetrates you. He's cool and "with it" enough to know that G-spots are a myth, G-strings are sexy and go ping when he tightens them around his penis, and the clitoris is sacred to women. He'll adore watching two women having oral sex and let you know how much he wishes you'd bring your dildo or sex toys to play every time you meet. He's bound to have a stack of sex manuals and latest gadgets in the boudoir, and no inhibitions about suggesting you make use of them. In fact, Mr. Aquarius has knowledge at his fingertips and penis tip; it's just his lack of emotional involvement that can make you feel like you're making love to a robot.

SEX IS SEX

Sex and love, well they're pretty complex issues for this cool customer. He does tend to make sex sound like a computer program, and tends to talk about shagging and bonking rather than "making love." But then again, he wants to rebel and do his own thing so you never know where you really stand or lie with him. He's a secret romantic but he won't let you know it. Usually he rabbits on about promiscuity and swapping partners, and how everyone should be free to have sex with anyone they choose, but he rarely does it himself. This man may seem unemotional, but he does have feelings. However, he'll keep them locked away from everyone, including himself. Sex is sex, and love? Well, that's for everyone, not just one other person.

HIS TOP TURNOFFS

SENSUALITY
He might try the odd oyster to check if it really lives up to its reputation as an aphrodisiac, but he won't want to fall about in silk sheets and massage oils.

COMMITMENT
Don't even think about it, let alone ask. The moment he thinks you might move in, he'll move on.

EMOTIONS
Leave them out of the bedroom. If you have feelings for him, discuss them like they are part of a scientific experiment, not something you own.

CONVENTION
If you're not willing to change the state of the nation or live in a beach hut, then this man will think you are totally boring.

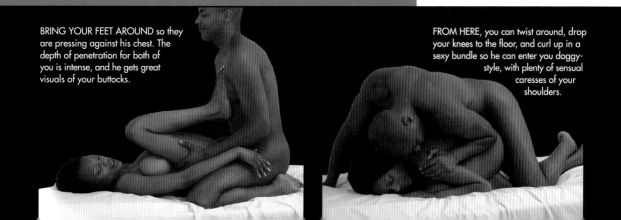

BRING YOUR FEET AROUND so they are pressing against his chest. The depth of penetration for both of you is intense, and he gets great visuals of your buttocks.

FROM HERE, you can twist around, drop your knees to the floor, and curl up in a sexy bundle so he can enter you doggy-style, with plenty of sensual caresses of your shoulders.

IS THIS THE ONE?

Not an easy catch, Aquarians need a friend (to add to their collection) rather than a long-term partner. But if you're as independent and free-thinking as they are, you could form a nonexclusive bond that is the nearest thing to love.

ARIES AND AQUARIUS

Aquarius is fascinated by Aries' impulsive nature but frequently prefers to observe rather than get involved. Good for experimental sex and long conversations into the night or a fling. But the ram's too hot and Aquarius just too cool.

TAURUS AND AQUARIUS

The bull is really too possessive for freedom-loving Aquarius. The water-bearer won't bear the bull's sensual indulgences for long, and the bull will get tired of all those exes who keep showing up for a free supper.

GEMINI AND AQUARIUS

You alternate between finding each other totally stimulating and totally frustrating. But you can develop a good long-term relationship based on friendship. A light-hearted approach to sex, but you could both stray too easily when apart.

CANCER AND AQUARIUS

Aquarius needs detachment; Cancer needs closeness. And although flattered by the crab's caring nature, it all gets too emotional in the sack. Once Aquarians have discovered the crab's sexual secrets, they'll want their freedom back.

LEO AND AQUARIUS

Aquarius believes in nonexclusive relationships, but Leo believes in utter exclusivity. Like any opposite signs of the zodiac, you have a feeling you're fated to be together, so this can be an exciting and dynamic physical rapport, for a while anyway.

VIRGO AND AQUARIUS

Both of you avoid emotional involvement. Stunningly different and therefore sexually addictive, but you both might just forget to talk about your feelings and hurt the other one unintentionally.

A fantastic physical rapport, based on **erotic mind games**. But Aquarius's **independent lifestyle** may conflict with Libra's need for a constant **companion**. Fantastic, sexy, **easy-going** relationship, not so simple for commitment.

LIBRA AND AQUARIUS

Often a **highly magnetic** and erotic relationship. But Scorpio wants **total involvement** and emotional intensity. Aquarius isn't interested in exclusivity or all those **feelings**. Great for an **unconventional** fling, if Scorpios can squish their jealousy.

SCORPIO AND AQUARIUS

Excellent for a **free-roaming** physical relationship. You both need oodles of **space** and dislike heavy-duty emotional scenes. You'll find each other mentally and **erotically stimulating**. A highly creative relationship for fun sex and long-term **laughs**.

SAGITTARIUS AND AQUARIUS

Very different needs. Capricorn wants a **conventional** lifestyle, and Aquarius prefers anything but. Yet a **lively**, ambitious sexual **adventure** for both, as long as Capricorn gives Aquarius space and Aquarius gives Capricorn a little **attention**.

CAPRICORN AND AQUARIUS

You share a **natural affinity** for the same physical and **mental pleasure**. Both of you approach relationships with a very **open mind**. Could be a great relationship, not particularly passionate, but completely **honest** and mutually **creative**.

AQUARIUS AND AQUARIUS

Aquarius's **radical belief system** and pride may jar with Pisces' more ephemeral **ideals**. Although physically it's all very arousing, you have very different **emotional needs**. Great for **romance** and a fling, but not easy long-term.

PISCES AND AQUARIUS

AND THE WINNER IS...

Aquarius identifies easily with the other air signs, Gemini and Libra, and probably will stay friends with them for life. But sexually, the water-bearer gets hooked on the water signs, particularly Scorpio, just because they seem to represent all those things Aquarians avoid in themselves, like emotions and feelings. However, if there is a long-term winner, then it has to be Sagittarius, who understands the wanderlust antics of Aquarius and knows that unconditional love works best.

LONG-TERM LOVE WITH AQUARIUS

Some signs of the zodiac naturally thrive on long-term relationships, but Aquarius believes in unconditional love rather than exclusive relating. If you talk about timescales—years, months, or even days—that implies you've already set conditions, and Aquarius is off. If you're as free-spirited as Aquarians, then they could be up for an unrestricted, open friendship.

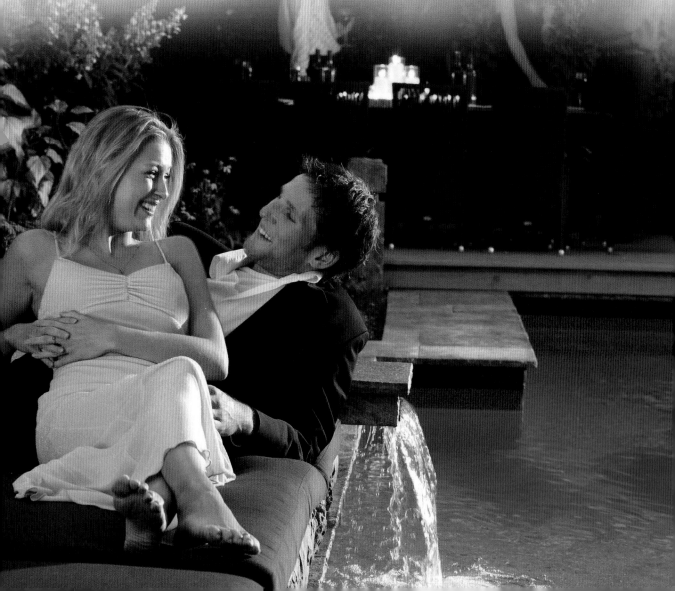

More than anything else, never show any signs of dependence on your Aquarian. Of course, they don't mind being asked their opinions or discussing the pros and cons of you buying a flat or living abroad. As long as you show that you're as self-reliant as they are, apart from needing help with the odd flat tire, then they'll begin to think that maybe you could be a friend for life. Long-term relating with Aquarius relies on one crucial thing: your willingness to be as altruistic and progressive about life and people as they are.

SEX IS NOT LOVE

Sex, as we've already noted, is sex to them. It rarely includes love in the equation. So if you're up for a sexy friendship, then remember that the Aquarian may have other sexy friendships too. If you're happy to share the water-bearer with the rest of the world, then your Aquarian is ready to share you too.

IDEALISTIC

Being idealists, Aquarians need support for their dreams, loads of personal space, and a good friend to chat with. The Aquarian dilemma is that they find it almost impossible to cope with their feelings and can't bear displays of emotions or jealousy in a partner. However, if you can be as rational and open-minded about life as they are, and discuss feelings objectively rather than let them show, then water-bearers will let you a little bit closer to that cool heart. It may be a long time coming, but if you can truly put your faith and belief in them, and subtly remind them that future civilizations depend on their visionary ideals, they may well decide you're about as perfect as anyone gets.

> Long-term love needs a **leap of faith**, but if it pays off, you'll be with one of the **brightest** and spontaneously **fun** signs around

UNBEARABLE

Aquarians don't actually believe in "dumping" anyone; they'd rather call it a parting of the ways. But if you really want Aquarius to bid you farewell, then simply turn into a waterspout and let loose with those messy emotions. Aquarians have a horror of being forced to accept that the emotional realm exists. They prefer to lead a cool, uncluttered life where everything is talked about rationally. So weep over your dinner, cry in public, stamp your feet, or show anger and your collected Aquarian will be off like a flash saving the whales instead of saving you.

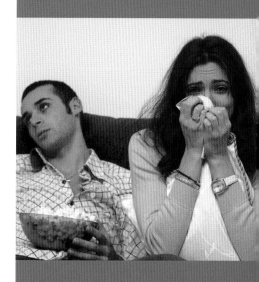

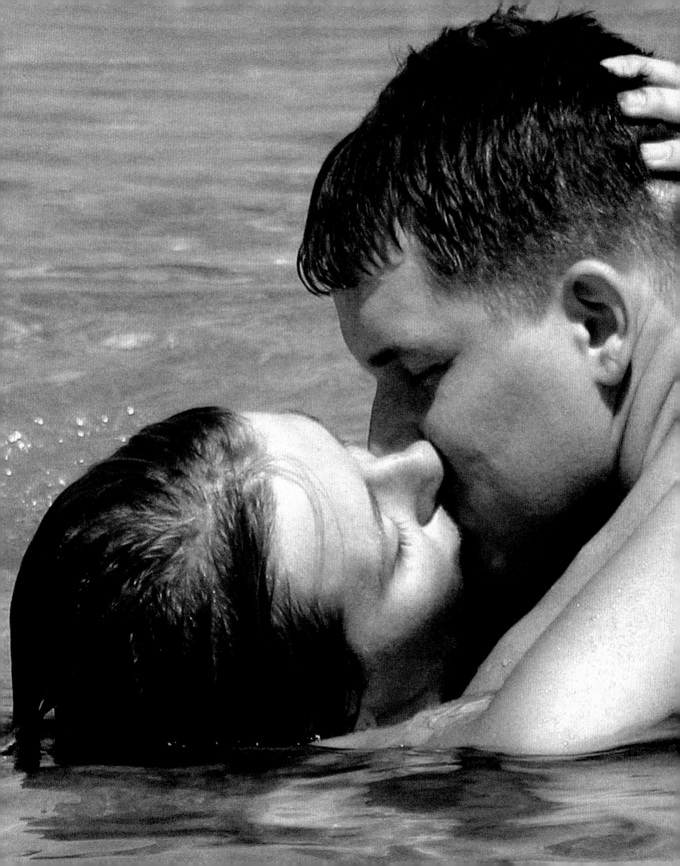

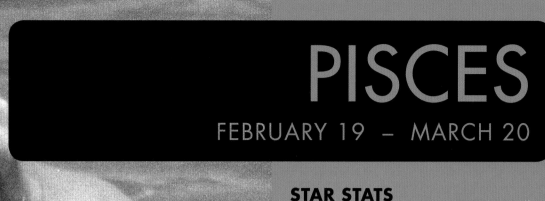

PISCES
FEBRUARY 19 – MARCH 20

STAR STATS

Ruling planet NEPTUNE
Signature symbol THE FISH
Metal TIN
Stone AMETHYST
Color LAVENDER

Where to find Pisces Hanging around wine bars, clubs, and pubs; can often be spotted daydreaming by the seashore or on some exotic beach.

Hot date Take Pisces to a champagne bar, then follow up with another surprise bottle of champagne under the moonlight.

Needs and desires Sensitive and dreamy, Pisceans need partners who can understand their changeable nature and desire for 24/7 romance.

Top turn-on Sex in the bath or the sea.

Sex positions ♀ The Dolphin
♂ Taking Turns

Sex toy Plastic water squirter.

Sex statistic 75 percent of Pisceans please their partners rather than themselves.

WHAT TO EXPECT WITH PISCES

There's something incredibly elusive and ethereal about the way Pisces enters your arms and then somehow disappears again. They want to be faithful but, because the fish are so seductive and easily led astray, they often get involved in superficial flings or one-night stands. Love and sex is everything to a Pisces.

Neptune—the planet of spiritual longing, romantic escapism, and self-sacrifice—rules Pisces. So it's not surprising that Pisceans have a problem with reality. And that includes the reality of their sexual identity. What is it? How can they really define it when it changes with every lover they meet? Somehow they fall in love too fast, play the role their lover wants them to play, and never really know what they truly want. But the sensual, mystical, and intuitive fish need to be needed and are dreamy, idealistic, and very dependent in a love relationship.

REELING IN THE FISH Pisces is easy to seduce with a flirty smile, but it may be harder to keep the fish's attention from roaming.

CHAMELEONS

Pisces is one of the most complex zodiac signs in love. The fish seem to embody a bit of each of the rest of the zodiac, merging with whoever they love and acting the role with ease. They will do anything for you: give up a job, romanticize about your future together, speak your language, and clean your car. In fact, Pisceans have a problem with boundaries and can get so involved in their partners' lives that they lose track of who they are themselves. They wriggle out of dates and are vague about their feelings, or their moods keep changing in an attempt to match yours. Chameleon-like and indecisive, they feel their sexual needs aren't as important as yours, which means they rarely please themselves. But their adaptable, easygoing attitude toward life and love makes them imaginative and magical lovers.

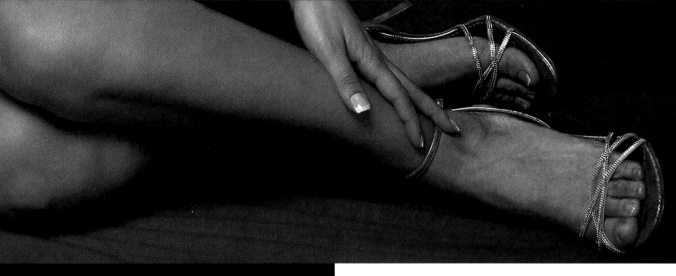

THE PISCES MAN

It's not so difficult to hook a Pisces; it's keeping him that's the problem. He's a social animal and loves to be surrounded by adoring women. You'll need to keep him entertained, have a fund of

> He's **easily** seduced by beauty, **romance,** or a "**come-on**" smile

fascinating anecdotes, and look like a princess. He's a tender lover, magical, funny, sexy, and elusive, but he falls in and out of love easily. The Pisces man is searching for something profound, but he's not exactly sure what it is. Tell him it's you.

THE PISCES WOMAN

The lady fish is as elusive as a mermaid. She'll be attracted by your looks, your sexiness, and what you can offer her, both romantically and materially. At best, you'll write love songs together, snuggle up in front of fires, and have sex all day long. She's so idealistic that weepy films, poetry, and phone calls feed her daydreams of romance. The lady fish falls in love often, and quickly. Seductive, escapist, and dreamy, she'll play whatever game you want to play. But remember, this mystical lady wants it all. She often breaks her lover's heart as well as her own and picks partners who disappoint because she's such an idealist. She's usually the last to see the reality of the relationship. Because she's willing to be what every man wants her to be, she pays a high price by sacrificing her real needs for the sake of emotional dependency.

PISCES IN A NUTSHELL

KEYWORDS Mystical; vulnerable; dreamy; impressionable; dependent; beautiful; romantic; escapist; elusive

LIKES Weepy films; music; art; candlelit dinners; acting; evasion

DISLIKES Direct confrontation; making decisions; reality

TRACKING DOWN YOUR PISCES

Pisceans are easy to find: they are usually hanging around in pubs and bars, and they absolutely adore socializing. Even though they may sometimes unexpectedly do a disappearing act, they'll magically appear again as if they've never left. Watch this space.

Pisceans are gifted with people and often end up as the office peacemaker or boss's confidante. They prefer a harmonious, low-key, pressure-free environment to work in. And if

to express all that talent through art, music, acting, or writing.

SOCIAL ANIMALS

Changeable and restless, Pisceans don't always follow

> Pisceans are never **happier** than when they're **letting go** of the **stress** and strains of the day in a bar surrounded by **friends**

there's tension or confrontation, they escape to the restroom or disappear to make the coffee. Pisceans will soothe bruised egos and campaign for peace, harmony, and goodwill in the office. Being psychic at times, they pick up feelings in the work environment and help anyone out in a crisis. Gregarious and fun to have around, they have powerful imaginations and need

up their dreams, and you can often spot them chattering away to others in their social circle about how their last partner didn't really know them or how they're misunderstood geniuses. The fish are definitely people people. But they are liable to get led astray by drugs and particularly alcohol, simply because it's easier than facing up to the responsibilities and duties they'd rather avoid in life. Party animals, they'll dance you off your feet, play and sing with the band, and enjoy wining and dining in romantic places.

WATERSPORTS

Piscean fish are, of course, naturally at home in water. They love swimming, water-skiing, and surfing. In fact, you'll track them down in seaside resorts, fishing on lakes, rowing gently down wide, meandering rivers, enjoying the delights of a spa holiday where they can be pampered, or lolling around on a float in the swimming pool. Check out those remote island vacations too. They love to get away from it all and gaze into the sunset across an empty beach. Go beachcombing and you have a good chance of bumping into a Pisces lounging around on the sand, or helping a crab to find its way home.

PLACES TO LOOK

THE LOCAL BAR

Pisceans still like to hang out with everyone else. And they prefer sitting at a bar stool where they can hear all the latest gossip.

ROCK CONCERTS/THEATER

All Pisceans have dreamed of being musicians or performers at some point in their lives. If they're not on that stage, they'll be behind it or bang in front of it.

WATER

If they're not gazing at it, they'll be in it. They are good swimmers, but lazy too, and might be the ones dabbling their toes in the surf rather than riding it.

ANIMAL RESCUE CENTERS

Pisces is a sucker for animals. And they really do care about lost dogs and cats, the plight of greyhounds, and rescued donkeys.

PISCES TOP TEN CAREERS

1 Musician
2 Photographer
3 Writer
4 Vet
5 Actress
6 Working with animals
7 Psychic healer
8 Secret agent
9 Social worker
10 Artist

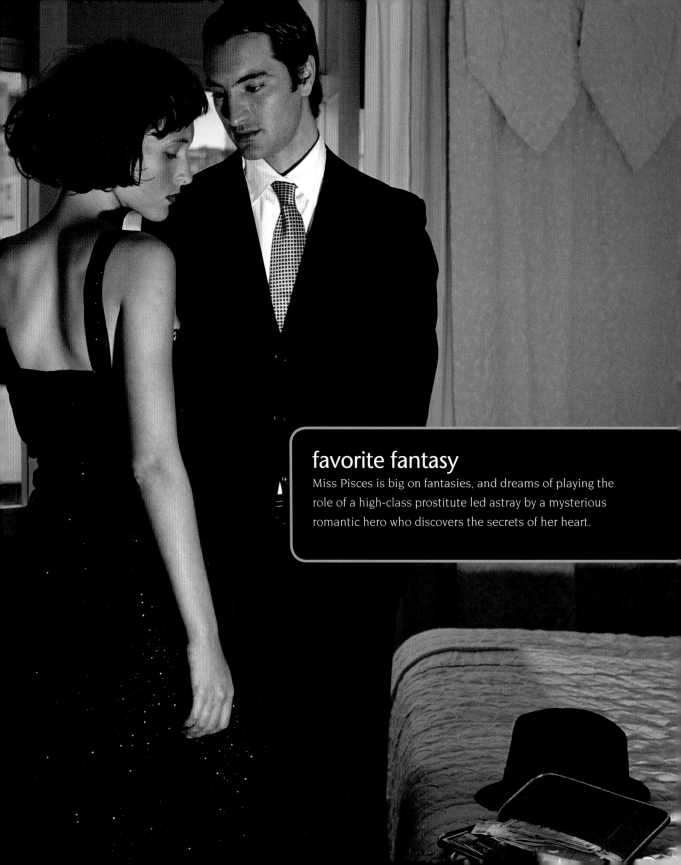

favorite fantasy

Miss Pisces is big on fantasies, and dreams of playing the role of a high-class prostitute led astray by a mysterious romantic hero who discovers the secrets of her heart.

WHAT WORKS FOR HER

Sensitive and acutely intuitive, the Pisces woman is a caring, tender, and sensual lover. She needs a complete merger of body, mind, and soul, and believes romance is sex, and sex is love. A sexual artist, she needs a lover whose passion and fantasies can blend with her own.

As for sex itself, well, that has to be an escapist experience. All sensual, romantic, and slow. The problem is she's so sensitive to your sexual needs that she often forgets or denies she has any of her own. A passive seductress, she enjoys being the submissive partner and letting you take the lead. She knows that passion and serenity don't always come in one male package. And the mermaid of the zodiac can carry on two love affairs at the same time so that she has a taste of both. Sometimes she hunts out men who are already involved or too hot to handle, knowing they'll leave her anyway. Pisces is always on a quest to seek her sexual soul mate, and her choice of partner is often mistaken in her search for the ideal man that she knows, deep down inside, doesn't exist.

> She's looking for **style**, gentleness, and **refinement**, but she also wants extremism and **dashing**, fiercely **passionate** sex

SPIRITUAL

She wants sex to be a spiritual experience, and she's so in touch with your sensual needs that her own orgasms are often withheld. Tantric sex could give her the chance to experience the ultimate erotic transformation.

HOW TO MAKE HER HORNY

Pisces is highly receptive to every move you make. But she needs to totally relax and have all her senses awakened to get truly aroused. The focus of her sexual energy flow begins in her toes as well as the soles of her feet. So concentrate on this potent astro-erogenous zone to bring this magical woman to the peak of sexual bliss. Nibble, suck, or lick her toes. Massage the soles of her feet, alternating between firm and light pressure to send her libido sky high. Pleasing you is a big part of her arousal, so for an erotic buzz, ask her to dip her toes into the cleft between your buttocks or to masturbate you with her feet. Then return the favor. She'll also adore it if you snuggle your body against hers from behind, and push the head of your penis through her thighs as you caress her clitoris.

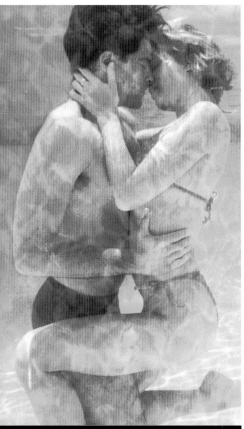

WATERBABE Miss Pisces is a bit of a sex mermaid beneath the water. You won't be able to resist leaping in at the deep end for your erotic enchantress.

SLOW AND SUBTLE

Her sexual expression is sensual, beguiling, and haunting. The mermaid's gift for slow arousal will lead you on a journey of sheer delight. She intuitively knows how to stimulate every nerve ending and every inch of your skin. But she does need emotional exchange in her lovemaking, and if you live in your head rather than your heart then she'll probably turn cold rather than hot. A truly feminine and subtle woman, she's instinctively tender and needs to be totally involved to feel pleasured and loved.

WATER BABE

Sensual, languid sex gives her the best adrenaline rush. Pisces is a water babe, so she usually enjoys being massaged and caressed underwater. Foreplay should be slow, languid, and intense, and her greatest erotic trigger is oral sex in water. Her nipples are also highly sensitive erogenous zones, so thrust your penis between her breasts and ask her to lick your freneleum as you push your penis up to her mouth. Buy water pistols, fill them with chamapagne, strip naked, and aim them at each other's buttocks or genitals. Then, when you're both soaking, lick her all over for bubbling arousal.

ROMANCE

Miss Pisces needs an expert lover, someone who's open about his fantasies, is not inhibited, and has passion and sensuality oozing from every bit of his body. She is very aware of "not being good enough" in bed, and she often learns every sex technique in the book, buys every sex toy available, or, in her youth, experiments with as many

THE DOLPHIN

Miss Pisces is sensitive to your sensual needs, so the Dolphin position offers you both a richly evocative sexual experience based on sexual and emotional closeness. You are in control of her movements, so this sequence requires a lot of trust between you. She prefers slow, languid arousal and anticipation of what is to come, so the build-up to sex is just as enjoyable for her as the act itself.

SHE HATES TO BE RUSHED, so take your time to build up her anticipation by whispering dirty fantasies into her ear while you caress her clitoris.

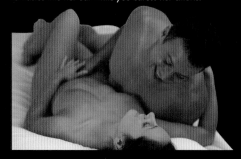

HER TOP TURNOFFS

VAIN MEN
She can't stand men doused in aftershave or beauty accessories. Leave the hair gel at home too.

FAST AND FURIOUS
Frantic lovemaking is one big yawn for her. She'll be wondering where her orgasm went, and won't be making a comeback.

BEING PUNCTUAL
She'll turn up eventually, but hates to be nailed to a time and place.

CLEARING UP
She's a romantic, so never ask her to clear away the empty glasses or make you breakfast.

SKEPTICS
If you don't believe in magic, angels, or astrology, then sorry, she won't believe in you.

men as possible. But it's not sex for the sake of sex, more that she's searching for her elusive soul mate. But sex should still be playful and exploratory.

She adores romantic films, fantasy, and evocative music. Unexpected romantic touches like roses on her doorstep, erotic text messages late at night, or a sexy phone call really turn her on. But she's also turned on by extremes and adores artists, poets, and victims of society, as well as shockingly dangerous or glamorous men. Pisces often plays the savior or the victim in a torrid relationship, which unconsciously gives her a big thrill because she can role-play and doesn't have to be herself.

Although Pisces has many fantasies, she steers clear of S&M, and certainly doesn't like indulging in threesomes or group sex. But she'll enjoy role-playing.

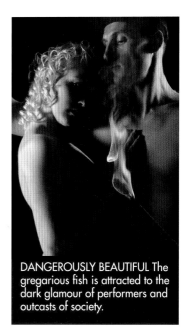

DANGEROUSLY BEAUTIFUL The gregarious fish is attracted to the dark glamour of performers and outcasts of society.

Anything from dressing up in high heels and suspender belts to playing a whore or a masked stranger. Public sex isn't her thing either, unless it happens to be a swimming pool, the sea, or secretly sharing a sauna, bath, or shower at a party.

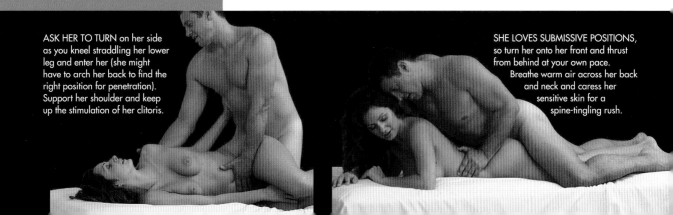

ASK HER TO TURN on her side as you kneel straddling her lower leg and enter her (she might have to arch her back to find the right position for penetration). Support her shoulder and keep up the stimulation of her clitoris.

SHE LOVES SUBMISSIVE POSITIONS, so turn her onto her front and thrust from behind at your own pace. Breathe warm air across her back and neck and caress her sensitive skin for a spine-tingling rush.

WHAT WORKS FOR HIM

Dreamy and sensitive, he doesn't quite know what he wants in a sexual relationship and prefers you to take the lead or dominate. Now that may sound like fun, but take care, because his libido is driven by a profound intuitive awareness of your needs and wants, so his often come second.

He's known for being a **bit of a rogue** when younger, and tends to fall in love **too fast** and leap in **at the deep end**

The fish is one of the most romantic and desirable of men; the only problem is that he can be downright elusive and hard to fathom. In fact, it's a bit of an art that he refines over the years to keep his potential soul mates guessing. After all, he's attracted to everyone around him, and falling for one woman does exclude all the other fish in the sea. But if you manage to catch this slippery but charming and sensual man, then he'll be the most imaginative, romantic, and magical of lovers.

SLIPPERY CUSTOMER

He seeks a profound erotic experience, but his sensitive side doesn't conform to current societal expectations that most men should be macho. So he can flip to extremes when you get beyond the kissing stage (and he does like the kissing stage), sometimes gentle, sensual, and poetic, the next moment playing the macho man or the passive victim. Watch out if he starts acting as though you are too demanding or possessive: he might just slip out the back door when you're not looking.

HOW TO MAKE HIM HORNY

The sign of Pisces rules the feet, and this is one of the most sensitive parts of his body apart from his nipples. Strangely, the sexual energy flow between the soles of his feet, his ankles, and up to his nipples is connected. So the sexual buzz will be intensified

back while you draw circles around his ankles and toes, massage his feet, then move sensuously up his body to kiss, suck, and nibble his nipples. He adores the feeling of your breasts brushing against his skin, so for the ultimate sexual treat, rub your breasts and nipples over his feet. Follow this up by using your breasts to slowly massage him all the way up his

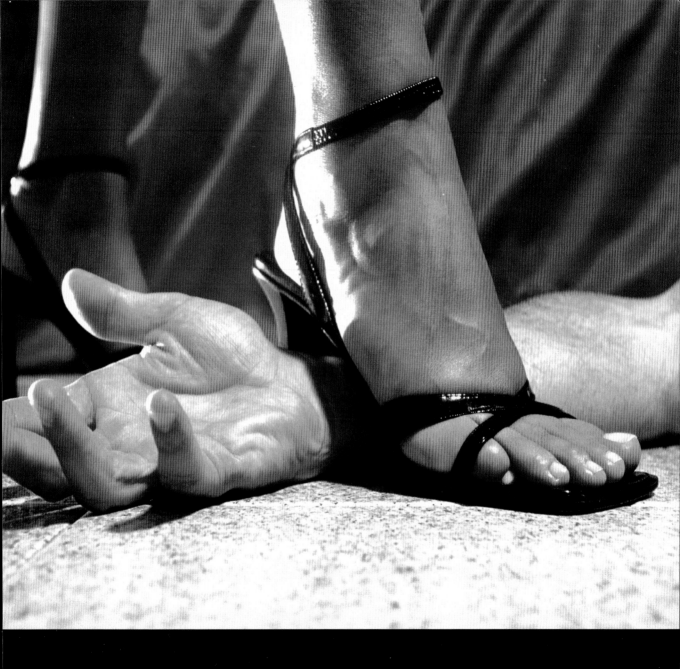

favorite fantasy

He likes the thought of being dominated by a strong woman
who will make him the sacrifice in her private cult of sexual
pleasure and literally walk all over him.

EAGER TO PLEASE

Mr. Pisces does, however, worry about his "performance." After all, the male social network goes on about the importance of "keeping it up all night," and "length." And, as you've probably guessed by now, Mr. Pisces isn't really that kind of macho man, so, for all his playful sexuality, he's acutely vulnerable about "doing it right." His own orgasm is often held back until he knows you're satisfied. But he's also got a pretty unreliable sex drive. If you try to pin him down to sex every morning or every night, he'll somehow avoid it or wriggle out of the occasion. Romance and ideal love are about the chase and the fantasy, and that's why his sexual habits are elusive and changeable: they're certainly not cageable, and he just won't want routine sex. He is instinctively gifted as a lover, but he does need variety, spontaneous lovemaking, and lots of romance. Be feminine, wily, and as elusive as he is; don't expect him to be on time on the first date; make sure you have good perfume, wine, and sexy underwear to keep his eyes fixed on you and you alone, and you might be in for a chance of a lifetime with this Neptunian dreamer.

ACTOR

Luckily, he adores role-playing and can be both the submissive youth and the dominant male. Ask him to be your sex slave for the day and give him time to indulge in his fantasy world. Because it is there, acting a part and drowning in a feast of romance and love, that he will eventually begin to discern what turns him on too, rather than just trying to please you. Sexual pleasure has to be a

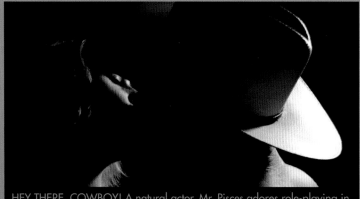

HEY THERE, COWBOY! A natural actor, Mr. Pisces adores role-playing in the bedroom, and can be anything from a dominant stud to Peter Pan.

TAKING TURNS

Mr. Pisces can be a little lazy in the sexual intercourse department. It's not that he doesn't have balls of fire; it's just that he likes the languid, sensual, slow approach. But he loves alternating between submissive and dominating positions. In this sequence you change roles and change angles for a sustained sex session. Pure pleasure of long-held arousal is more important to this man than the orgasm.

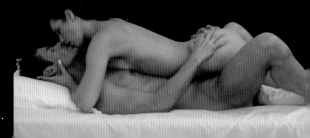

INDULGE HIS SUBMISSIVE SIDE by starting off in the Missionary position with you on top. You can take full control of things with your hip movements and ease him into action.

mutual thing or this man won't be around for long.

He's aroused in romantic settings, so opt for candlelit dinners at home with plenty of aphrodisiacs, like strawberries, champagne, oysters, or avocados. Feed him with your fingers, or

ORAL FIXATION

Oral sex is one of his favorite pastimes. Give him oral sex while he's sleeping or first thing in the morning to really wake him up. Ask him to kneel in front of you while you are standing up—preferably still

HIS TOP TURNOFFS

EXPLANATIONS

Never insist that Pisces explains his feelings, motives, or behavior. He simply can't rationalize why he does what he does.

JEALOUSY

If you're the green-eyed type, stay away. The fish is one of the most gregarious and flirtatious of men and needs to play, not be worked on by you.

> He's **uncannily** aware of exactly what **turns you on**, so let him **dominate** whenever he wants

lips or ask him to drip wine or juice over your breasts and nipples and lick it slowly off. Video yourself wearing sexy lingerie, and seductively explain what you would like to do with him in bed. Watch it together, then do something completely different to what you suggested— he's turned on by surprises.

wearing a dress, somewhere discreet but in a semipublic location. Water sex is a great way to sneakily get him to do the things you love best, so take a bath or shower together. Ask him to masturbate you with the lather or bubbles, bring him to the brink with your tongue and mouth, then slip on top of him.

STRAIGHT ANSWERS

Ask him outright if he loves you and he'll tell you tomorrow is another story. Badger him and he'll run away forever.

MATERIALISM

Show more interest in your latest outfit than his line of poetry and he'll write you off his love list.

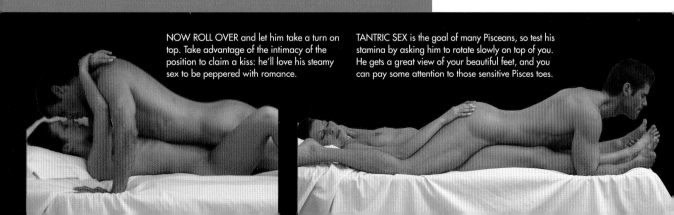

NOW ROLL OVER and let him take a turn on top. Take advantage of the intimacy of the position to claim a kiss: he'll love his steamy sex to be peppered with romance.

TANTRIC SEX is the goal of many Pisceans, so test his stamina by asking him to rotate slowly on top of you. He gets a great view of your beautiful feet, and you can pay some attention to those sensitive Pisces toes.

IS THIS THE ONE?

Pisceans, for all their evasiveness about commitment, make superb long-term lovers once they fall in love. Kind, considerate, and romantic, the dreamers of the zodiac need someone to truly empathize with their idealistic dream worlds.

ARIES AND PISCES

Brimming with passion and audacity, the ram can't resist the fish's lush sensuality. And Pisces easily surrenders to the games and uninhibited sexual style of the ram. Difficulties could arise when Pisces wanders and Aries is away crusading.

TAURUS AND PISCES

The bull is always drawn toward Pisces' sensitive nature and intuitive talents. Pisceans are fascinated by Taurean's down-to-earth approach to life, and feel safe in their hands. Can be an eye-opening love affair for both, but not easy long-term.

GEMINI AND PISCES

You are both able to adapt to each other's changeable and restless natures. Pisces will drift along easily with the rather inconsistent sex drive of Gemini, and you can both indulge in each other's fantasies too. Can be a long-term success.

CANCER AND PISCES

Pisces knows how to please you, and you know what goes on behind the role-playing. Both of you are sensitive and highly intuitive about how the other feels, so you don't have to explain your unpredictable moods. A very private and sexy bond.

LEO AND PISCES

Pisces prefers to escape into a dream world; Leo would rather be the only fantasy in Pisces' life. Superb sexual rapport—sensual, magnetic, and lush—but in the real world, basically a difficult relationship.

VIRGO AND PISCES

Natural opposites in the zodiac, somehow you're a devoted duo. You have tense then teasing moments, insatiable and unstoppable. Arousal between you is profound; excellent prospects for long-term sexual rapport.

You can both escape into fantasy, dreams, and sex. Pisces is looking for the ultimate experience; Libra for the perfect one. Romantic and sexually exotic, but imagination may not be enough to keep you together when life's practicalities kick in.

LIBRA AND PISCES

The fish is a social animal and prefers to roam and gossip. Scorpios are discreet and hate their intimate life broadcast around town. Good for sexual affinity, but lifestyle needs are very different.

SCORPIO AND PISCES

The archer is a bit of a sexual roamer while Pisces adores clandestine romance, so they might meet through a love triangle. A wonderful sexual rapport if you give each other room. Great for spontaneity; hard to keep a track of each other.

SAGITTARIUS AND PISCES

Capricorn may fall under Pisces' sexual spell for a while, but not an easy relationship between you. Pisces has a desire for the unusual, the unknown, and change, but these are all things that Capricorn loathes.

CAPRICORN AND PISCES

Aquarius's radical belief system and pride may jar with Pisces' more ephemeral ideals. Although physically it's all very arousing, you have very different emotional needs. Great for romance and a fling, but not easy long-term.

AQUARIUS AND PISCES

Trapped in a fantasy world, you both rarely look outside at the reality. A totally erotic rapport, but your dependency on one another grows too easily. This may result in one of you acting the martyr through fear of abandonment.

PISCES AND PISCES

AND THE WINNER IS...

Undeniably, Pisces has an easy rapport with the other mutable signs, Gemini and Sagittarius. Especially in the sack, where the dynamic is

are also good bets to keep Pisces romantically amused and inspired. But for long-term success, Cancerians probably win by a mile, simply because they understand the longings and confusions of the Pisces soul, and their warm hearts and gentle ways

LONG-TERM LOVE WITH PISCES

Pisceans have difficulty in committing themselves to only one person, simply because there are so many attractive and beautiful people in the world, and they all seem to offer something special. Deep down the fish wants to merge in a deeply emotional and spiritual bond, but it's the reality of working at relationships that leads them into difficulty.

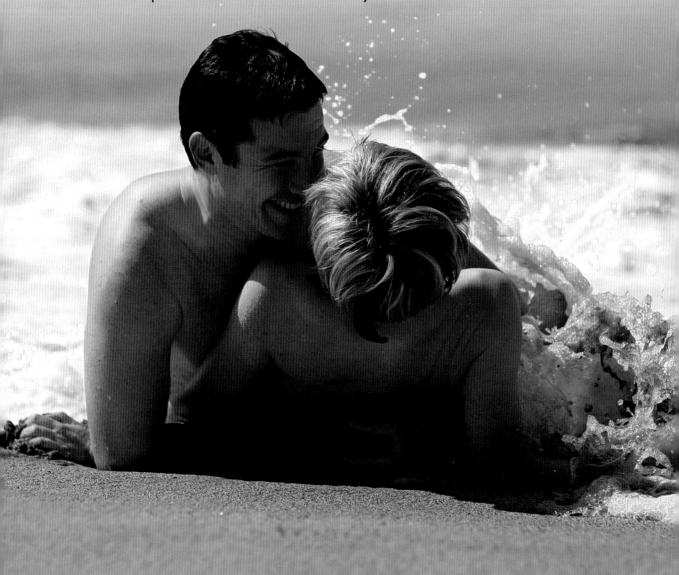

Understand the Piscean need to go off in a dream, to surf their lonely waves and yet be a social animal, and you'll probably last longer than most. If you have an independent lifestyle, don't try to push the fish around, nag, or complain, then they'll be loyal and true. Learning to live with Pisces isn't easy if you're a controlling, pragmatic type. They'll probably like having you around for a while if you make their decisions for them. But

enigmatic and keep them guessing what you're up to. If you're looking for a conventional relationship, stay away.

COMPASSIONATE

Pisces lives in a dream world, preferring to dwell on shades of gray rather than black-and-white facts. If you're logical and ultrarational, think carefully whether you can cope with this without shattering their fantasies. Respect their restless nature,

> Be the magical, **inspirational, fun-loving** person that Pisces can **trust**, and your fish will prove **trustworthy** too

Pisces doesn't like being forced to do anything and prefers to be guided rather than led, so diplomacy and tact work best.

MYSTERY

Your best bet for long-term love is to give them their space and have your own too, but always be there to provide practical advice when they ask for it. Pisces thrives on mystery, so remain a little aloof and

support and help them ground their extraordinary artistic talents, and Pisceans will reward you with compassion and sensitivity. They're not the most stable of people: their feelings are ever-changing, and they don't like to be pinned down. But if you're happy to go with the flow of their moods, and side with their romantic aspirations and dreams, then you could be the one to keep the fish hooked for life.

SLIPPERY CUSTOMER

Pisces hates confrontation, and also doesn't like being told what to do. So if you want them to dump you, you're going to have to be ultradogmatic and upfront with it. Be dictatorial around the home, give them grief about where they go and who they see, and make it clear that you're going to chain them to you forever. You'll soon find that your slippery Pisces customer will simply slide away from you into the ocean in search of some other more laid-back fish in the sea.

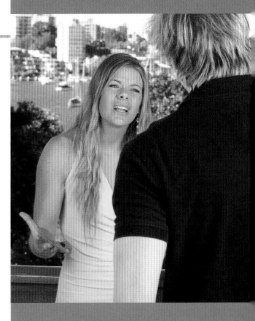

SEX GRID

Use this at-a-glance guide to discover the relationship dynamics of any sun-sign combination. Each pair of sun-signs create a unique sexual energy flow, which might be a "conversation stopper" or "sensual and dreamy."

	Aries	Taurus	Gemini	Cancer	Leo
Aries	Fiery pulse-raiser	Spicy body warmer	Conversation stopper	Sensual and steamy	Flamboyant and hilarious
Taurus	Spicy body warmer	Spicy and sensual	Earthy sexual-booster	Steamy and indulgent	Passionate pulse-raiser
Gemini	Conversation stopper	Earthy sexual-booster	Double the fun	Steamy and challenging	Lighthearted and liberating
Cancer	Sensual and steamy	Steamy and indulgent	Steamy and challenging	Close and cuddly	Steamy and passionate
Leo	Flamboyant and hilarious	Passionate pulse-raiser	Lighthearted and liberating	Steamy and passionate	Fiery and provocative
Virgo	Cool, potent buzz	Earthy delight	Wicked merger	Sensitive affinity	Luscious and laid-back
Libra	Adrena-line-pumper	Hot and responsive	Teasing and romantic	Dreamy and escapist	Romantic pulse-raiser
Scorpio	Hypnotic but teasing	Sensual energy-booster	Intensely competitive	Deeply erotic fantasies	Steamy and passionate
Sagittarius	Nonstop adventure	Sexy differences	Liberating pulse-raiser	Exhausting but magnetic	Exhilarating adventure
Capricorn	Intense energy-booster	Sensually addictive	Slow tension build-up	Challenging libido booster	Competitive and ambitious
Aquarius	Red-hot challenge	Erotic and compelling	Pacey with highs and lows	Cool but demanding	Experimental and liberating
Pisces	Pulsatingly sensual	Spicy rapport	Demandingly sensual	Super-erotic arouser	Sexy, uneven energy

HOW TO USE THE CHART

Simply look down the column of signs on the left for the one you want to find, and then run your finger across the horizontal column at the top until you find the other sign you're looking for. Where they meet in the grid are several keywords for the sexual dynamics of those two signs. For example, say you're a Virgo and your lover is a Libra. Look on the left-hand side column for Virgo, then along the top line for Pisces, and the square where they meet in the grid says your relationship will be "sensual and romantic."

Virgo	Libra	Scorpio	Sagittarius	Capricorn	Aquarius	Pisces
Cool, potent buzz	Adrena-line-pumper	Hypnotic but teasing	Nonstop adventure	Intense energy-booster	Red-hot challenge	Pulsatingly sensual
Earthy delight	Hot and responsive	Sensual energy-booster	Sexy differences	Sensually addictive	Erotic and compelling	Spicy rapport
Wicked merger	Teasing and romantic	Intensely competitive	Liberating pulse-raiser	Slow tension build-up	Racey with highs and lows	Demandingly sensual
Sensitive affinity	Dreamy and escapist	Deeply erotic fantasies	Exhausting but magnetic	Challenging libido booster	Cool but demanding	Super-erotic arouser
Luscious and laid-back	Romantic pulse-raiser	Steamy and passionate	Exhilarating adventure	Competitive and ambitious	Experimental and liberating	Sexy, uneven energy
Erotic and earthy	Sensual and romantic	Exciting and challenging	Hot responses	Earthy and indulgent	Sensually fascinating	Perfect pulse-raiser
Sensual and romantic	Laid-back and sensual	Wickedly fascinating	Sublime sensual libido-booster	Erotic but demanding	Racey and orgasmic	Sensual and dreamy
Exciting and challenging	Wickedly fascinating	Volatile and erotic	Passionate pulse-raiser	Torrid and hypnotic	Wicked libido-pumper	Escapist fantasy
Hot responses	Sublime sensual libido-booster	Passionate pulse-raiser	Irresistible pulse-raiser	Fiery and buzzing	Unpredictable and exciting	Electrifying and hot
Earthy and indulgent	Erotic but demanding	Torrid and hypnotic	Fiery and buzzing	Earthy erotic bliss	Earthy but experimental	Romantic and indulgent
Sensually fascinating	Racey and orgasmic	Wicked libido-pumper	Unpredictable and exciting	Earthy but experimental	Delicious tension build-up	Intensely arousing
Perfect pulse-raiser	Sensual and dreamy	Escapist fantasy	Electrifying and hot	Romantic and indulgent	Intensely arousing	Idealistic and dreamy

WHAT THE FUTURE HOLDS

We all want to know what's going to happen to us a few weeks from now, or even a few years ahead. We all spend time dreaming about what we might be, without really thinking about who we are in the present. But with awareness of your good and bad qualities, needs, and desires, you can take responsibility for your destiny. It's all about changing the aspects of yourself that make you difficult to live with or that hold you back from finding true love.

This section won't predict your future for you. In fact, it's asking you to start being creative with it. After all, it's your future, and no one else's, isn't it? The future is something that you can control and influence if you learn more about yourself. And astrology tells you all about who you are. Carl Jung said that "a man's life is characteristic of himself." In other words, our emotions, talents, and drives attract similar experiences or kindred people along our life journey. Armed with astrological self-awareness, you can make choices that lead you to the future you truly want. The more unaware of who you are, the more you will feel fated in life. The more aware of who you are, the more you can maximize your innate potential and discover the kind of relationships that are right for you.

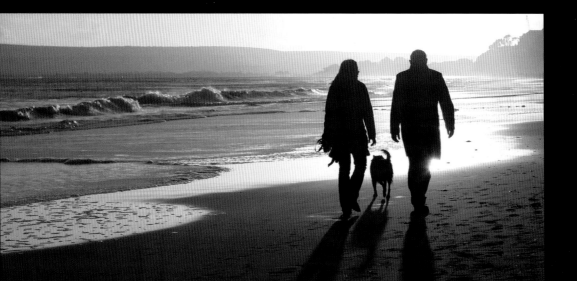

ARIES

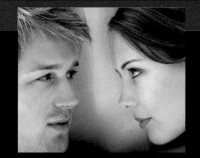

You have **strength**, guts, and a powerful sex drive, so choose partners who accept that you have a **"warrior" image** to live up to. But do remember to show your **softer**, sensual side as well. Your desire for a more **adventurous** relationship will be met if you make your **true needs** clear. Be **less self-centered**, and then you'll achieve the **passionate** affair you're seeking.

TAURUS

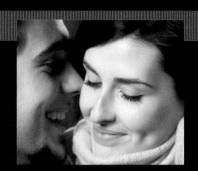

You can have a truly **beautiful future** if you give your lover some **space**. Be less possessive, show more **trust,** and don't feel embarrassed about your **sensualist** nature. Rather than calculating **every move** in the relationship game, listen to your partners and let them make their **own decisions**. Being **less controlling** will bring you happiness and reward your senses.

GEMINI

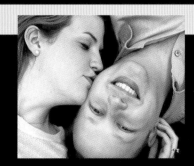

You're so **lighthearted** your lover just doesn't know where he or she **stands** with you sometimes. So you need to learn to be more **sensitive**. Ask how your partner feels and show you care. You have feelings too, so honor your **inner desires** and **don't pretend** to be someone you're not. You'll soon be on a sexual roller coaster, with sensual **thrills** and romantic **highs**.

CANCER

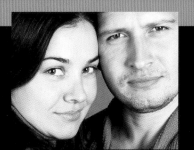

It's easy to take a **backseat** and imagine that love is always going to pass you by. But however **insecure** you feel, you have to put the past behind you and **move forward** on the path of true love you secretly **long for**. If you sit on the sidelines, you'll simply **regret** missing those chances. Your emotional future is **in your hands**, so dump any emotional baggage and move on.

LEO

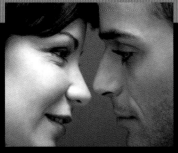

It's true that you're all **fire and brimstone**, but in the future you need to learn to value a little **caution**. Challenging relationships are **inspiring**, but you need to see where you're heading first. Whether it's a physical, intellectual, or **emotional journey**, your destiny will be everything you want it to be. If you can learn to **love yourself**, so can someone else.

VIRGO

Don't fear change, but go with its **magical flow** in love matters and you'll develop a greater sense of personal **security**. It's time to **free yourself** from the chains of other people's expectations, and create your own set of **rules about love**. Let yourself be more **spontaneous** in love. Seduce someone before you have time to write down the pros and cons. It will be **liberating**.

LIBRA

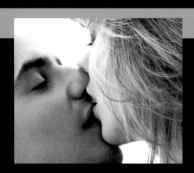

Physical desire is wonderful and natural, but love has other facets too. Don't be swayed just by a **beautiful face** or the **glamour** of someone's lifestyle. Develop your **self-esteem** rather than squish it. You will soon be walking those **romantic pathways** to a deeper involvement. So **show off your IQ**, but don't forget that your **feelings** have a place too.

SCORPIO

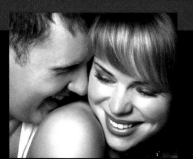

Your focus needs to be how to **negotiate** and **articulate your desires** and feelings rather than excommunicate them. Those **emotional drawbridges** between you and a lover can be lowered. And you'll discover complete **bliss** in your **reenergized** sense of harmony. A deeper commitment will mean you can at last experience the **closeness** you crave.

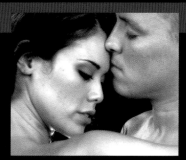

Romance isn't just scoring points over the restaurant table; it's about being a little cool and elusive. So, on the road ahead, try to use your imagination, be more tactful, play the game your partner's way too, and your sex life will dramatically change for the better. Either you'll meet the lover of your dreams or your current relationship will take on a whole new sensual meaning.

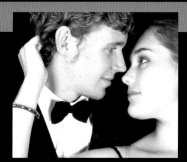

Love isn't just about hard work: it requires passion and fun too. So aim to chill out, take the odd risk, and don't fear your instincts. Try leaping in at the deep end to revitalize your sexual spirit. Be less defensive about your feelings and laugh about love rather than try to contain it. Then you'll create the happiness you truly seek in any relationship.

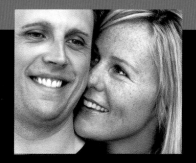

Free yourself from the judgements you make about every potential lover and be less controlling about your feelings. Analyze carefully if you really want to commit to only one person, as your desire for freedom is equally strong. Learn to be as compassionate toward yourself as you are toward everyone else, and you'll discover true, unconditional love.

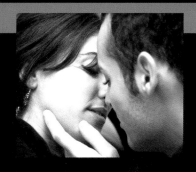

You need to learn to ask for what you want, sexually and emotionally. Remind yourself that you deserve love because you're you, unique and special. When you find out how to balance your romantic ideals with life's practicalities, then inner harmony will bring outer success. Take as much as you give, and you'll discover you can go your own way and find sexual contentment.

MOONSTRUCK

If you've read through your sun-sign description and feel it doesn't sound like you, it may be the effects of your natal Moon are particularly potent right now. The Moon in your birth chart influences your reactions, secret needs, and emotions, whereas the Sun influences your actions, desires, conscious intentions, and personality. At times in your life, you'll identify with the Moon in your chart rather than the Sun, because our emotional side takes over from our rational, conscious nature when we're in very stressful circumstances or complex relationships. See if you recognize yourself in the overview below. If you don't know your moon-sign, you can contact me on my website www.sarahbartlett.com and I'll let you know what it is for free.

MOON IN ARIES	YOU REACT impulsively, without thinking of the consequences. If your lover doesn't call, you'll charge to his or her place for a showdown.	YOU NEED a challenging partner and oodles of physical contact, but your independence is vital for your emotional wellbeing. Sexually, you have to be the center of attention, but you don't like to feel emotionally tied to anyone.
MOON IN TAURUS	YOU REACT slowly. You hate being pushed for answers, and you're always in control of your feelings. You dislike change and find security in the familiar.	YOU NEED a close, cozy relationship and a lover who makes romantic gestures every day. You feel possessive about your partners, and if they want to change something like their hairstyle, you'll seduce them into keeping it the way it was when you first met them!
MOON IN GEMINI	YOU REACT to situations with quick wit and clever conversation. Your lover has to be as intellectually bright as you, or you get bored quickly.	YOU NEED a friend first, a lover second. Love must be unconditional, and rarely do you let anyone know what your true feelings are. Lighthearted and gregarious, you're nurtured through new ideas, while your sexual curiosity knows no bounds.
MOON IN CANCER	YOU REACT unpredictably. If your lover is delayed, you'll imagine the worst; if he or she admits to missing you, you'll pretend you don't care.	YOU NEED loads of hugs and kisses, not just sex, to feel really secure. You're acutely vulnerable and your cool streak is just a cover-up for your sensitive heart. Your feelings are so changeable that your partner can't work out the real you.
MOON IN LEO	YOU REACT like a true drama queen (male or female!). In fact, you expect to be treated like royalty, so if you're not, you'll stamp your feet.	YOU NEED to be under the glare of the spotlight and in control of the relationship with a glamorous partner to match. Intensely individualistic, you're nurtured by a sexually exciting relationship and a lover who won't take you for granted.

YOU REACT rationally and calmly. If your partner forgets to call you, you'll think of all the possible reasons why he or she hasn't, and opt for the most sensible solution.

YOU NEED an intelligent lover and someone who doesn't make emotional demands on you. Your feelings are well hidden, and passion makes you nervous. If you do ever admit to feeling anything, you really mean it.

MOON IN VIRGO

YOU REACT in a very passive way. In fact, you often compromise too much and loathe voicing an opinion simply because you don't want to cause a scene.

YOU NEED peace at any cost. If there's any whiff of emotional theatrics, you'll be out of the door in a flash. As long as your relationship is romantic and harmonious, you're happy, but you also need a large social circle to keep you amused.

MOON IN LIBRA

YOU REACT by exercising that infamous sting in your tail. Acutely manipulative, you can make your partner believe he or she is in the wrong, even when you are!

YOU NEED a powerfully sexual relationship where you can totally trust your lover. When you fall in love, it's a serious, intense business. You are very aware of your feelings and can become obsessed with knowing what your partner is feeling too.

MOON IN SCORPIO

YOU REACT impetuously, without thinking of the consequences. What you do best is make light of things; what you do worst is promise the earth when you don't mean it.

YOU NEED loads of personal freedom and lively, fun-loving, sexy companionship. Fiery and self-motivated, you feel nurtured in a no-strings relationship, and if anyone tries to emotionally tie you down, you'll run in the other direction.

MOON IN SAGITTARIUS

YOU REACT cautiously. You'll take your time to work out whether it's worth your while to go on a date with X, or if there's anything to be gained from it in the future.

YOU NEED emotional honesty and a partner who is looking for a bonding sexual relationship. You're wary of those chaotic feelings inside yourself, and you don't open up easily. Secretly vulnerable, you have one of the kindest hearts around.

MOON IN CAPRICORN

YOU REACT by being as awkward as possible. You always react in a way that's not expected of you, just to make life interesting. Emotions don't come into the equation at all.

YOU NEED a quirky, sexy relationship with no strings. You thrive on intellectual stimulation and friendship first and foremost, and you're nurtured by talking about feelings in general rather than feeling them for yourself.

MOON IN AQUARIUS

YOU REACT in a charming and seductive way. Endlessly forgiving, you hate creating scenes, and you want to be the best lover in the universe.

YOU NEED a dreamy, romantic relationship where you don't have to make decisions. You have no emotional boundaries, which means you can merge with your lover but can also get led astray by the wrong type or sacrifice your goals for your partner.

MOON IN PISCES

INDEX

PHOTO CREDITS

The publisher would like to thank the following for their kind permission to reproduce their photographs:

Key: a = above, b = bottom/below; c = center, l = left; r = right; rh = running header; t = top

Abbreviations: SS = Shutterstock; GI = Getty Images; PDC = Photos.com

002-003 SS/lev dolgachov; 004tr, 15 SS/Pedro Talens Masip; 004cra, 33 SS/Pedro Talens Masip; 004crb, 51 SS/Pedro Talens Masip; 004br, 69 SS/ Pedro Talens Masip; 005tl, 87 SS/Pedro Talens Masip; 005cla, 105 SS/Pedro Talens Masip; 005clb, 123 SS/Pedro Talens Masip; 005bl, 141 SS/Pedro Talens Masip; 005tr, 159 SS/Pedro Talens Masip; 005cra, 177 SS/Pedro Talens Masip; 005crb, 195 SS/Pedro Talens Masip; 005br, 213 SS/Pedro Talens Masip; 006–007 GI/Samantha Messens; 008–009 GI/altrendo images; 010-011 GI/Ghislain & Marie David de Lossy; 013cl SS/Juha Sompinmäki; 013cr SS/Carly Rose Hennigan; 013bl SS/Galyna Andrushko; 013br SS/Joel Kempson; 014-015 PDC; 016bl; GI/Photographer's Choice; 017t GI/April; 018–019 SS/Nelson Hale; 020 SS/Vova Pomortzeff; 022tl GI/PicturePress; 023tr GI/PicturePress; 025 PDC; 026tl GI/Stuart McClymont; 028–029 SS/lev dolgachov; 030b PDC; 031br GI/Jonathan Storey; 032–033 GI/Ebby May; 034bl SS/Iryna Kurhan; 035t SS/1418336 Ontario Ltd; 036–037 GI/Ranald Mackechnie; 038 GI/ Thomas Hoeffgen; 040l SS/Graca Victoria; 041tr SS/MANDY GODBEHEAR; 043 SS/Scott Bowlin; 044cl SS/ Niserin; 046–047 SS/Iryna Kurhan; 048b SS/vgstudio; 049br SS/Inger Anne Hulbækdal; 050–051 SS/Najin; 052bl PDC; 053t SS/lev dolgachov; 054–055 PDC; 056 GI/Jason Hetherington; 058tl SS/Gabriel Openshaw; 059tr SS/Z. Adam; 061 GI/ David Perry; 062cl SS/lev dolgachov; 064–065 SS/Tad Denson; 066l PDC; 067br SS/ lev dolgachov; 068–069 SS/Carl Durocher; 070bl GI/Eryk Fitkau; 072–073 PDC; 074 SS/Kiselev Andrey Valerevich; 076tl GI/Eryk Fitkau; 077tr PDC; 079 GI/Holly Harris; 080tr SS/Ana Blazic; 082–083 SS/Najin; 084b GI/ altrendo images; 085br SS/Phil Date; 086–087 GI/Laureen Middley; 088bl GI/Britt Erlanson; 089t PDC; 090–091 GI/ Chev Wilkinson; 092 GI/David Perry; 094tl GI/Ebby May; 095tr SS/lev dolgachov; 097 GI/DreamPictures; 098tl PDC; 100–101 SS/Alex James Bramwell; 102b PDC; 103br SS/ Bobby Deal/RealDealPhoto; 104–105 GI/Eryk Fitkau; 106br PDC; 107t PDC; 108–109 SS/bora ucak; 110 GI/David Perry; 112tl SS/Carl Durocher; 113tr SS/ISM; 115 GI/ James Martin; 116cl PDC; 118–119 PDC; 120b PDC; 121br PDC; 122–123 SS/Iryna Kurhan; 124bl SS/Zsolt Nyulaszi; 125t PDC; 126–127 PDC; 128t GI/altrendo images; 130tr GI/April; 133 GI/Hans Neleman; 134tl SS/lev dolgachov; 136–137 PDC; 138br PDC; 139br SS/Phil Date; 140–141 SS/vgstudio; 142bl SS/Adam Radosavljevic; 143t SS/lev dolgachov; 144–145 SS/Nsilcock; 146 SS/William Frederick Lawson; 148tl PDC; 151 GI/Stephen Stickler; 152cl GI/Leslie Lyons; 154–155 SS/vgstudio; 156b SS/ vgstudio; 157br SS/Sladjan Lukic; 158–159 SS/Yuri Arcurs; 160bl PDC; 161t GI/altrendo images; 162–163 PDC; 164 GI/Tony Hutchings; 166tl GI/John Davis; 167tr PDC; 169 SS/vgstudio; 170cl GI/April; 172–173 SS/MaleWitch; 174b PDC; 175br PDC; 176–177 GI/Ghislain & Marie David de Lossy; 178bl SS/Diego Cervo; 179t SS/lev dolgachov; 180–181 SS/Bartosz Ostrowski; 182 GI/John Davis; 184tl SS/Adam Radosavljevic; 185tr SS/Nici Kuehl; 187 GI/Howard Kingsnorth; 188tl SS/vgstudio; 190–191 SS/Dewayne Flowers; 192br SS/CW Lawrence; 193br SS/ Alex Brosa; 194–195 GI/April; 196bl SS/Luc Beziat; 197t GI/Barnaby Hall; 198–199 PDC; 200 GI/Garry Wade; 202tl GI/Luc Beziat; 203tr SS/1418336 Ontario Ltd; 205 SS/PhotoSmart; 206tl GI/Robert Daly; 208–209 SS/ Wallenrock; 210b PDC; 211br SS/Diego Cervo; 212–213 SS/Zdorov Kirill Vladimirovich; 214bl SS/Mark E. Stout; 215t SS/Jorge Cubells Biela; 216–217 SS/Steve Lovegrove; 218 GI/Martin Sanmiguel; 220tl GI/Larry Gatz; 221tr SS/ Filipchuk Oleg Vladimirovich; 223t GI/altrendo images; 224cl SS/Chris Rabkin; 226–227 SS/Alex James Bramwell; 228 SS/Galina Barskaya; 229br SS/Nicholas Sutcliffe; 230–231 SS/Vova Pomortzeff; 232b SS/Joe Gough; 233tr SS/Yuri Arcurs; 233cra SS/vgstudio; 233crb SS/Jeff Thrower (WebThrower); 233br SS/Raisa Kanareva; 234tl SS/Diego Cervo; 234cla SS/lev dolgachov; 234clb SS/lev dolgachov; 234bl SS/Iryna Kurhan; 235tr SS/Tad Denson; 235cra SS/Wikus Otto; 235crb SS/Dana Burns; 235bl SS/ Diego Cervo; 236–237 SS/Lena Grottling
All positions photography: Jeremy Hopley
Jacket images: front SS/Darren Green; back SS/Iryna Kurhan